Automated Insulin Delivery

How artificial pancreas "closed loop" systems can aid you in living with diabetes

DANA M. LEWIS

v 0.0.6

DEDICATION

For everyone living with diabetes -
and anyone who loves and supports someone with diabetes

CONTENTS

DANA M. LEWIS

DISCLAIMER

It probably goes without saying, but it's always worth noting as you dive into this book or any of its content: I'm not a medical doctor. I'm a person with diabetes who's been living with it for 19(+) years. I've helped to build & encourage adoption of DIY and other kinds of APS technology. I've used it myself now for more than 7 years. I'm biased. And I'm human.

The technology & approaches discussed in this book may not be approved by a regulatory body in your country. However, whether you're considering DIY or other APS technology, or *any* approach to managing your diabetes: I hope you'll evaluate it carefully and decide what works for you. Talk with your doctor or healthcare team if you're considering making any changes.

Also, your diabetes will vary. It will vary from mine and everyone else's. When you read stories, advice, or suggestions, either in a book or on the Internet or elsewhere - please remember that. What works for one person may not work for you, and that's ok!

PREFACE: MY STORY AND THE
EVOLUTION OF DIY CLOSED LOOPING

The room was dark and still, but I couldn't move a muscle.
I had woken up for some reason, but I realized I could not move.
Had someone broken into my apartment? Was I paralyzed with
instinctual fear? No, all was quiet and there was no movement.
Instead, the realization dawned that my blood sugar was probably
low. I managed to turn my head slightly to the left, and somehow
could see the screen on the receiver of my CGM. It said the worst
thing it could possibly say: "LOW". That meant my blood glucose
(BG) levels were below 40 mg/dL, and likely dropping.

I could also see the juice box sitting right there on the
bedside table. I needed to grab it, take the straw off and open the
wrapper, and manage to get the straw in and take a drink. Four or
five simple steps. I had done so thousands of times in my decade
of living with type 1 diabetes. So why wasn't I doing it now? Why
couldn't I move? Why was I paralyzed? If I didn't drink the juice,
my blood sugar might keep dropping and I could slip into a coma

and die. Since I lived alone, it might take days for someone to notice that I had not shown up to the office or was not responding online. I was going to die, and this was what it felt like to be afraid, alone, and in the dark unable to move.

And then I woke up.

Thankfully, that was "just" a terrible nightmare. However, it's the nightmare that changed my life - and I may even be bold enough to say that it ultimately changed the lives of thousands of other people with type 1 diabetes, too.

****

The day after I had that terrible nightmare, I remember staying in my office at work until around 9pm. I had called my parents, who were in Alabama, from my office in Seattle. I was crying. I was afraid to go home, because I didn't want to go to sleep. I was afraid of what might happen if that nightmare became reality. Because unfortunately, it could happen. Although uncommon, and numbers on actual incidence are difficult to find (because it's hard to know what causes it), the phenomenon known as "dead in bed" from type 1 diabetes can happen. There's a variety of reasons it may happen, which I'll describe later. On that night in March 2013, it didn't matter to me how unlikely it was to happen. It felt very, very likely to happen and very real.

Some of the solutions at the time would have involved getting a roommate. I didn't want a roommate. I had lived with roommates in the dorm throughout college, and I was thrilled to have moved to Seattle for work, and be living by myself. Getting a roommate felt like a step backward.

The best solution I had do at the time was what I had already been using for years. Every night before bed, I texted my mom to tell her when I expected to be up or get going for the day, such as when my first meeting was. Every morning, my mom (who was in a time zone two hours ahead of me), would text me around the time I was planning to get up. The plan was that if I didn't respond after a while, she would call me. There were numerous reasons I might not have responded right away, such as if I had gone in to work early or got wrapped up in a spontaneous meeting. Or, in the worst case, that I hadn't woken up to my phone alarm because my blood sugar was too low. Ideally, I would answer the phone or text her back and let her know I was awake, ok, and fine. But the plan was that if she couldn't reach me by phone, she would then call the apartment manager of my building and have them come check on me. If they couldn't get me to come to the door, they'd call 911.

Thankfully, up to that point (and even until now), 911 never had to be called. It seemed, and seems, so silly to need all of these backup plans when there's an even more simple solution: making the alarms on my continuous glucose monitor (CGM) alarm louder.

****

To just about anyone who's not living with a chronic disease, this problem seems easily solvable. Change the alarm on the CGM. Allow users to configure the alarm sound, so they don't get used to always hearing the same sound, and their brain will be less likely to ignore the sound.

However, changing a medical device is a lot harder than you might think. Devices are designed many years before they actually come to market. Making a change to a device often takes half a decade or longer. Despite speaking to all of the CGM manufacturers on the market many times, and begging them - in person, on the phone, and by email - to enable users to make the alarms louder… it didn't do any good.

To be fair, they did respond, but the companies' responses were frustrating. I was told that they were working on it and it would be out in the future. (Although louder alarm options have never come to market on a hardware-based device). I was told that it wasn't a problem for most people. (At the time of this writing, there are 45,000 search results on Google when one types in "louder CGM alarm", with a variety of hacks and tips proposed . Even in 2013, I definitely wasn't the only one with this concern.)

That answer also didn't feel like it was enough. I was frustrated by being told to wait. I was living with the problem then, that day, that night, and every night for the rest of my life. And what could I do about it? Nothing. I was "just" the patient and the "user" or "consumer" of the device, with no option to change medical devices to better suit my needs.

****

In April 2013, I began dating Scott Leibrand. On our first date, when we began talking about type 1 diabetes, he asked why my CGM didn't talk to my insulin pump. Coming from a tech background, he (and everyone else who doesn't have chronic illnesses and hasn't become used to the weird status quo of healthcare technology being antiquated, and devices not being interoperable with each other) didn't think that made very much sense. But again, we couldn't do anything about it. I told him about my nightmare, and my idea for a louder alarm system that would send alerts to my phone, instead of relying on the physical CGM device. It would be designed to be loud, and with varying types of sounds, to wake me up. But if I didn't wake up, it would then alarm my mom or someone else and give them the earliest possible warning to call and check on me.

There was one flaw with this idea: it required accessing the CGM data in real time, and at the time, there was no real-time data sharing from any CGM device. In fact, I couldn't even get my own data off my physical CGM. The FDA-approved software was only approved for PC computers - and I had a Mac. So not only was real-time data a pipe dream, but so was personal review of my data from my own device. It was frustrating, to say the least.

****

Fast forward a few months later. I had been active on Twitter for years, and somehow saw a tweet surface by a gentleman named John Costik. It showed a picture of how he was somehow managing to pull the CGM data off the receiver - and in real time! He was then sending it to the cloud, where he could view his son's data remotely. I was thrilled - if we could manage to do the same thing, we could then build my louder alarm system!

I sent that tweet to Scott, who suggested that we actually reach out to John and ask him to share his code, so we didn't have to recreate the wheel. This was new territory for me - my professional background is in communications, so I was unfamiliar with the concepts of "open source" and people freely sharing their code to help one another. Scott messaged John, and John said yes, he would share the code. I was thrilled!

At the time, pulling data off the CGM still required a PC, so I borrowed an old, clunky PC laptop from Scott to sit under my bedside table. We set up John's code so that when I plugged in my CGM into the laptop, it would pull the data off the receiver. There was a script that would tell it to pull the data off every 5 minutes, when a new BG data point would come in. Scott and I designed it to add the BG data to a file in the Dropbox folder on the computer. It would then be uploaded to the cloud, and downloaded to a virtual Linux server we set up for the purpose. From there, we designed a simple series of rules to tell the computer when to alarm me. We also got a simple $5 alarm app called "Pushover", which would receive the commands and send the alarms to my phone.

DIYPS

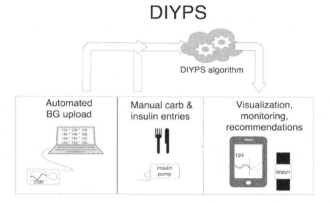

It worked fantastically, even on the first night. I got several alarms telling me that my blood glucose level was going high, or low. And I actually heard the alarms! It was an incredible relief to know that I had this backup system in place.

As I had envisioned months ago, I also wanted to build a tiered alarm system, in case I still somehow managed to sleep through the alarms while I was deeply sleeping, or if my BG was exceptionally low. Scott and I put together a very simple webpage to display the data. We also added simple web buttons. When I woke up to an alarm, I would open my phone and press the "snooze" button. This would snooze the system. However, if I didn't respond to my alarm in a period of time, and if my blood glucose reached a certain level, it would then alarm the next person. (At this point, I decided to have Scott be the recipient of the next level of alarms, instead of my mom, since he was co-designing the system, and also because he lived 20 miles away.)

The tiered alarm system worked well, too. A few days after

we created it, Scott got alarmed, woke up, and called me. I woke up to his phone call even though I had slept through the Pushover alarm. I was able to drink a juice box and go back to bed safely.

After that, we decided that we should add more buttons to the system. Instead of just hitting a "snooze" alarm, we designed and inserted a few buttons for the key actions I usually was taking: eating carbs (i.e. drinking a juice box or eating a snack), taking insulin (if my BG was high), or setting a short, temporary basal rate of 0 for 30 minutes (effectively reducing my insulin temporarily to ward off a future dip in BGs). That way, Scott would be able to see not only that I was awake, but also what treatment, if any, I had done.

I became an exceptionally well-trained guinea pig (in my own words), pressing a button every time I ate something or adjusted my insulin delivery. We realized that, in addition to real-time CGM data, it would be valuable to combine all of the manual inputs along with the CGM data in order to forecast into the future what was likely to happen. This meant that I could get *predictive* alarms and alerts - instead of just reacting to already low or high BG levels.

We used the publicly available data on insulin activity curves to simulate the predicted insulin activity for correction boluses to bring down high blood sugar. But we had also noticed that withholding normal basal insulin caused blood sugar to rise, so we decided to track *net* insulin activity to model this insulin reduction. This means that you could actually have "negative" insulin activity, compared to your normal baseline levels of insulin activity from your basal rates. Having "negative" insulin-on-board (IOB) meant that there would be the opposite effect of positive insulin on board: blood sugar would rise from having less insulin than usual. This is helpful because you can't remove insulin after it's been injected or infused into your body. However, you can reduce your baseline amount of insulin to help compensate for insulin you've already received, and help reduce or even prevent blood sugar from dropping low in the near future.

This was a huge step forward. Within a few months, we had evolved from a simple, "louder alarm system" to essentially having built an algorithm and an "open loop system" that suggested insulin dosing adjustments and carb corrections. We didn't know it at the time, but this was the precursor to the first open source closed loop algorithm that would later be known as OpenAPS.

****

We jokingly called this system "DIYPS", which stood for the "Do-It-Yourself Pancreas System". It was life-changing.

I no longer feared going to sleep at night. If my BG was predicted to go low or high, or was actually low or high, it would alarm me. If I didn't respond to my alarm, it alarmed Scott, and he would call me.

Over the few months that we were creating DIYPS and were using it at night by my bed, Kevin Lee and others also used John's code as well. Kevin in particular spent a lot of time making an Android-based phone uploader, so that you could have a mobile phone upload the CGM data to the cloud. This enabled me to plug my CGM receiver into a small Android phone instead of the larger stationary PC, and use DIYPS throughout the day. It helped immensely during the day, too.

One day I had eaten lunch, taken insulin, and left for my next meeting. However, I found out that the meeting had been moved to another campus - about a mile away. I had to walk, quickly, to make it to the meeting. My insulin from lunch started to take effect even more quickly, due to the exercise. DIYPS pushed an alert to me in the middle of my hurried walk, and I drank a juice along the way. As a result, I didn't have a nasty low BG when I arrived at my meeting.

I was enamored. And I had a feeling that this type of tool could help other people too. I began talking about it online & sharing with other people. Scott and I were invited to participate in DiabetesMine's D-Data Exchange in June 2014.

This event was notable for us for two key reasons. First, we got to have a table during the "demo" portion, and talk to people about DIYPS. I was excited to share with other people what we had done, how it was working for us, and our ideas to safely share it with others. We had used John's code to get data off the CGM, which is how I learned about open source. I wanted to make DIYPS open source, too.

However, during the demo discussions, a few people came up and were asking us about DIYPS. How did it work? We were making dosing recommendations off a CGM? Did we know that the CGM was not designed for that? As we answered their questions, we learned that these were individuals from the FDA (the U.S. regulatory agency with oversight for medical devices). The end of that conversation involved a strong recommendation to *not* share or distribute the code for DIYPS, because among other reasons, it was making dosing recommendations from a CGM, which wasn't yet approved for that. And regardless, they considered sharing code to be distributing medical devices, which would be regulated by the FDA.

Gulp. Sharing code on the internet was seen as distributing a medical device? That didn't make sense to us, but we respected (and were scared by) the input. After all, we were two individuals who developed something that worked for me. We didn't want to get sued, or have a US Marshal come and kick down my door, because we shared our code online.

But the other reason that D-Data 2014 was notable was meeting the gentleman with the demo table to our left: Ben West. Ben was showing off years of his work, figuring out how to reverse engineer and evaluate the communications from an insulin pump. We didn't recognize it yet at that very moment, but his work was and still is pivotal in the movement of open source closed loop insulin delivery.

We walked away from D-Data re-evaluating how we would be able to share DIYPS. At the very least, we knew we could talk about the concept, even if we didn't share the code of DIYPS itself. I could raise awareness for the problem of not-loud-enough CGM alarms and the lack of customization.

****

Over the next few months, we talked with more people about DIYPS, and learned more about Ben's work. One day - we can't remember exactly when - a collective lightbulb went off. Ben's work included not just the ability to read from the insulin pump, but he had also discovered the commands to talk and "write" to the insulin pump. Those commands included being able to set temporary basal rates on the pump remotely, using the Carelink USB stick (designed to read data from the pump) and a computer. What if we used a computer holding our DIYPS algorithm, and translated the "recommendations" into commands, and sent those commands to the pump? We could close the loop?

We could close the loop.

****

That was late fall in 2014. We had a chance to present DIYPS more formally at the fall D-Data Exchange in November. We explained DIYPS, what we had learned from it, and what we wanted to do next. We shared that we thought we could close the loop, and that we would try to do so.

We joked about setting a deadline for August 2015 for closing the loop. Why then? Well, Scott and I had gotten engaged, and would be getting married in August 2015. That meant he would be married to me - and all my CGM alarms! So by the time we got married & moved in together, Scott was very invested in figuring out more diabetes automation, because he knew he was the lighter sleeper, and the one most likely to wake up to those alarms!

I always mention our "goal" timeline because I'm blown away by how fast we actually managed to close the loop. Granted, we had already developed the algorithm (for DIYPS), and I had spent a year testing, tweaking and improving it. Ben had spent years figuring out the pump communications. Yet within three weeks, Ben, Scott, and I had managed to put together a combination of systems where the DIYPS algorithm would output recommendations that were sent as commands that the radio stick would send to the pump. The data would be read off of the pump, and the CGM, on a regular basis. The algorithm would update the calculations and the predictions, and do it over and over again.

I very clearly remember the moment that we were able to send a command to the pump. It wasn't connected to my body - we were testing with a spare pump - but the circle appeared on the screen that alerted us to the fact that a temporary basal rate had been successfully sent to the pump. A few days later we managed to fully close the loop. The night that we closed the loop, I decided to test it on the pump connected to my body. I felt very confident in doing so, because I had the alarms on my CGM as well as the supplementary (and very loud) phone alarms that we had designed. Originally, I planned to wake up every few hours to monitor the system, but I love to sleep, so I decided I would just sleep and not bother about the monitoring.

I woke up the next morning and felt discombobulated for a minute. Why did I feel different? Oh yes, I had let the closed loop system run. I took a look at my CGM, and was astonished to see that my BGs had stayed in range all night. I didn't have a single alarm go off! Anytime my blood glucose rose, the closed loop system gave a little more insulin. When my blood glucose level dropped and was predicted to go low, it reduced the baseline insulin accordingly. My discombobulated feeling wasn't that anything was wrong - it was the fact that I had gotten a solid 9+ hours of sleep with my blood glucose perfectly in range, and without having to wake up at all.

At that point, I surprised Scott. We originally planned for this to be an overnight-only system that would just sit on my bedside table. However, it was working so well, I wanted to see what it would do during the day, too! I put it in my laptop bag with one of Scott's spare batteries, and went to work.

You probably won't be surprised to learn it worked well during the day, too. It sat on my desk at work, or was in my bag or pocket when I walked around town. I never wanted to turn it off or let anyone take it from me. In fact, four and a half years later, the only time I have not looped was when I was forced to stop, one weekend soon after I had started. I had corrupted the SD card on the Raspberry Pi mini-computer I was using due to unplugging and replugging the power source so many times as I moved between work and home, and letting the battery die a few times. The system stopped working on a Friday afternoon, and we couldn't find anywhere to get an SD card faster than Amazon Prime 2-day shipping, so I had to go from Friday afternoon until Monday afternoon without my closed loop. It was terrible going back to my old normal. The brief downtime was such a clear reinforcement of how much benefit this closed loop system was providing me, both day and night. We got the SD card replaced and I have been using a DIY closed loop (with many more backups) ever since.

****

DIY closed looping worked incredibly well for me. The computer sent commands to the pump via the radio stick, telling the pump to set or adjust 30-minute temporary basal rates to adjust my insulin delivery. If the system broke or died for any reason, then at the end of the 30-minute temporary rate, it would fall back to "standard" pumping, just like before. We also knew it wasn't if, but when and how, the system would fail, so we designed it to fail safely. We *assumed* that the system would fail, so we designed the system to only set a temporary basal rate if it would be safe to let that basal run to completion and then revert back to standard basal rates. Insulin delivery was adjusted conservatively with that assumption that each adjustment was the last command the system might send.

We wanted to find a way to share this with others. We didn't think a lot of people would want to do it, but a few might. And we had spent so many months improving the algorithm, and designing for safety. We thought it was important for others to be able to start from the point we had reached, rather than recreate the wheel and re-learn some of the same safety lessons.

However, we vividly remembered the conversations with the FDA employees who said that DIYPS code sharing would be 'distributing a class III medical device' - and DIYPS at that time was just a system that made recommendations. Now we were wanting to share code for a system that would allow people to automate their insulin delivery.

We also felt a moral imperative to share what we had learned. Many people who are unfamiliar with type 1 diabetes think that an automated insulin delivery system introduces many new risks. And it does. However, the calculation *also* must include the everyday risks of living with type 1 diabetes. It's already incredibly risky. Insulin is a life-saving drug, but too much insulin, or the right amount of insulin given at the wrong time, can cause harm, or death. Insufficient insulin can also cause issues in the long run. Having a computer track insulin dosing every five minutes and make micro-adjustments limited by software and hardware safety limits is, for most of us, a lot safer than doing things manually.

We decided that we would share what we had learned, but we'd take additional measures in order to share it as safely as possible. First, we wrote a plain-language 'reference design' that discussed the system's safety design and outlined all the safety considerations built in via both hardware and software. This documentation would be the recommended first stop and first read for anyone considering building themselves a similar system. Second, we would share the code components that had been built individually. There were two distinct pieces. One was the 'openaps toolkit', which was all of the separate commands to read and write to a connected insulin pump. The other eventually became the "oref0" repository, which included the actual algorithm that would determine the needed insulin adjustment. So, the code in and of itself was not a single device. No one would press a single button and "get" a pancreas. You would have to take all the components and build it yourself. We decided to call this project, and the movement, "OpenAPS", to stand for the 'open source artificial pancreas system'. OpenAPS was launched on the web on February 4, 2015.

FOREWORD BY AARON KOWALSKI

Making a difference and improving lives – there are few goals more satisfying and powerful. Since starting at JDRF, I've been fortunate to have participated in a transformation that has occurred over the last decade or so and is now a global focus for me. This revolution has improved the lives of thousands of people around the world – including my brother and me – and has challenged the status quo. It's an honor to write a foreword to this book and for a true visionary – Dana Lewis – who has and continues to make a massive difference in the field of diabetes and has improved thousands of lives playing a pivotal role in a key component of this revolution: the mainstreaming of do-it-yourself (DIY) automation of insulin delivery.

In 2018, I was invited to speak to the employees at a large diabetes company and two children and one young adult spoke beside me to the group about the challenges of living with type 1 diabetes. During the Q&A an employee asked the young woman what it was like to go through high school with T1D and she began to cry. She noted that she was bullied for having diabetes and that had caused her to stop dosing insulin when needed at lunch and other times, and ultimately to completely hide her diabetes. Her glucose levels careened to dangerously high levels and she had to withdraw from school. Fortunately, she has recovered but was scarred by the experience. I highlight this story because it so painfully and succinctly crystallizes the underappreciated aspects of diabetes management, and a huge unmet need for people with diabetes. That is – diabetes is more than glucose control! Diabetes is stress, it's anxiety, it's sleep, it's stigma, it's carbohydrates, it's family dynamics, as Dana describes it is fear of hypoglycemia ... and it's impossibly variable. For years I've been arguing that diabetes treatments must address both sides of the equation – glucose control and quality of life. Dana and her now-husband Scott saw this and have developed a solution that finally does that: and the response from users has been incredible!

Now, you may be asking why the former lead of the JDRF Artificial Pancreas (AP) Project would be touting DIY systems (actually I hope that you aren't, but will address the question nonetheless!). It's because DIY and commercial systems are not mutually exclusive! JDRF has deployed significant resources to speed the development and availability of AP or automated insulin-delivery systems (AID systems). I'm thrilled that Medtronic launched the 670G and have a number of colleagues and friends benefitting from that system tremendously. Having Beta Bionics, Bigfoot, Diabeloop, Insulet, Roche, Tandem, Tidepool, and others developing systems is wonderful. That said, having a robust DIY ecosystem has been a tremendous addition to the space. The hashtag that crystalizes the sentiment in the community is #WeAreNotWaiting. We needed these solutions years ago, not years from now. The DIY community took the bull by the horns, integrated their medical devices with cell phones and watches and other non-medical technologies, and began to rapidly iterate on problems and develop and evolve solutions that added value to them – the community. These solutions address both sides of the equation – they improve glucose control and they reduce the burden of diabetes management!

I must confess that when Dana and Scott told me that they were going to launch OpenAPS that I urged caution. This was despite seeing countless hours of study data demonstrating the safety and efficacy of hybrid closed-loop systems in outpatient real-world clinical trials. But patients developing, testing, and sharing their own systems was uncharted territory and a bit scary! However, what Dana, the DIY community and many people with diabetes will tell you – and I fully agree – is that living with type 1 diabetes, day in and day out, and being your own control system is scary too. The data supports that. In the JDRF CGM trial[1], the average person in the trial spent nearly 10 hours a day above 180mg/dL and over an hour every single day below 70mg/dL, even with significant work and effort (the other side of the equation!) [2]. Hypoglycemia – every single day! The T1D Exchange

---

[1] Juvenile Diabetes Research Foundation Continuous Glucose Monitoring Study Group. Continuous glucose monitoring and intensive treatment of type 1 diabetes. N Engl J Med. 2008; 359:1464-76. Epub 2008 Sep 8.
[2] Foster et al. State of Type 1 Diabetes Management and Outcomes from the T1D Exchange in 2016-2018. Diabetes Technol Ther. 2019;21:66-72. Epub 2019 Jan 18.

has shown this quantitatively as well. Unfortunately, severe hypoglycemia is still much too common. Living with diabetes – even with a CGM and a pump – is still very difficult and better tools are needed.

AP systems are not a cure for diabetes. They still require site changes, CGM changes, tweaking and, particularly early in their use, some patience. That said, as Dana points out throughout and in the "Success Stories" chapter – the results can be transformative. My own experience is just that. I use a DIY AP system and can't imagine how I did it before. Despite nearly 35 years of T1D experience and having worked in diabetes for nearly 15 years it's still a very hard disease to manage! The impact of an APS system in my life has been less hypoglycemia, a better A1c, less work to get there, and most impactful – better sleep. The near normalized overnight glucose levels never get old. It's the first time that both sides of the equation have been improved simultaneously for me – better glycemic control and better quality of life.

Congratulations Dana for making such an impact. DIY AP systems are improving people's lives for the better. This book is an incredibly comprehensive view of how we got here, what these systems are, considerations on potential use, and a detailed view of what to expect if you do adopt an AP system (DIY or commercial). I often say that diabetes is a club that we don't want anyone to join. But, you will find some incredible people in this club. Dana and Scott are two such people. So are the countless others who have contributed to the development of novel ways to help people with diabetes. The connectivity and technological advances enabling

APS are amazing. JDRF remains committed to one day seeing cures for T1D alleviating the need to wear devices and dose insulin. In the meantime, we need better tools to help people to achieve better outcomes – both improving glucose levels as well as easing diabetes management burden. It's amazing to see this happening so rapidly today.

Aaron J. Kowalski, PhD
JDRF President and CEO
Co-founder of JDRF Artificial Pancreas Project
T1D Dx 1984, Brother T1D Dx 1977

INTRODUCTION

OpenAPS was the first open source do-it-yourself artificial pancreas system, but is not the only one. You'll learn more throughout the book about different DIY systems, their similarities and differences, and how they compare to various commercial systems.

At this point in time (now 2021, in an updated version of the book), there are estimated to be thousands of individuals worldwide who've chosen to use DIY closed loop systems over the last four years. People choose to use them for different reasons. Some people, like me, choose it for better and safer overnights with type 1 diabetes (you can read more about my story in the preface). Other people want to improve their A1c or time spent in range. Others want to reduce the cognitive or physical burden of work required to achieve their goals.

Some people may choose to continue using DIY, and others may choose to switch to a commercial system in the future. There will be a growing number of commercial closed loop options in the future, too. It's exciting to have so many choices becoming available for people with diabetes. Just like traditional insulin pumps, though, they will all have different features and options, including different hardware and different algorithms. What works well for one person may not be the right choice for another person.

Whether we're talking about DIY or commercial, it's important to remember that a closed loop is not a cure for diabetes. These systems can work incredibly well, reduce burden and improve outcomes for people living with type 1 diabetes. But just like switching from MDI to an insulin pump, it takes work. There is a learning curve.

I've learned a lot from my personal use of OpenAPS over the last four and a half years. I've also learned a lot through helping, and observing, other people's journeys in using DIY and more recently, also commercial versions, of artificial pancreas systems. I've spent a lot of time writing tips, tricks, and suggestions for people over the years. Although this content has been fully available online for years on my blog (www.DIYPS.org), I recently realized that most people thinking about looping in various forms don't have a single place to get a comprehensive picture about their technology options, the lessons the community has learned about the learning curve of switching from manual to automated insulin delivery, and a straightforward, plain-language explanation to guide them in making their choices.

My hope with this book is to share these lessons learned, and provide a guide to help people consider what's important for them to choose the system that best works for them and their lifestyle. With the information shared in this book, I hope you'll feel more informed, and empowered, in your choices related to closed loop technology, and have insight into what your learning curve will look like.

HOW TO GET THE MOST OUT OF THIS BOOK

As I mentioned, some of this content has been available for years. However, I've completely re-written it all and added around 25,000 words of new information to help guide people in understanding and switching to automated insulin delivery. I want this content to be easily accessible to people. So I've chosen the following formats for the content:

1. **A traditional, physical "book" format (what you're reading now!)** - a physical, printed book that's available through self-publishing. It's priced so that every 2 copies purchased will fund an author-priced copy that I will donate to hospitals, libraries, etc.

2. **An "e-book" format** - a version that can be downloaded to your Kindle, from Amazon.

3. **A PDF format** - which you can download and read on your computer or other e-reader of choice. This is accessible   at http://www.artificialpancreasbook.com/download

4. **A website** - so you can review portions of the content anytime, and see any changes over time. There will also be

additional links and videos with more content. The website and its content are open source, so if you see any typos or have suggestions, you can make those suggestions or edits directly! www.artificialpancreasbook.com

The PDF and web versions of this book are free, but if you have found value in any of the content (or similar content that I've written at DIYPS.org over the past five years), please consider using the donate button if you didn't buy a physical or Kindle copy. Any funds received will be used to buy more author-priced copies to be donated, or be donated to my charity of choice, Life for a Child. Or, feel free to make a donation to Life for a Child directly! Thank you.

The open-source web version will drive subsequent edits and updates to the other three formats (PDF, e-book, and physical copies), and I'll keep a version history page on the website so if you purchase the book, you can look and see what's changed over time in each of the versions or formats.

This book won't have everything, though. It's the beginning of the tip of the iceberg of all the knowledge and wisdom that is out there in the diabetes community. So if you find yourself reading this and saying "I know all of this, but it's missing XXX" or "I wish the book talked more about YYY" - great! Please, do go to your blog and write more of what you think is missing, make edits and additions to community documentation, or make edit requests and suggestions for additions to this book. The more people we have sharing their knowledge, the more people will be able to learn! I'm also happy to share what I've learned about the self-publishing process for e-books and physical books. If this has inspired you to write your own book, and you have questions, please don't hesitate to reach out.

1. WHAT'S A CLOSED LOOP OR ARTIFICIAL PANCREAS SYSTEM, AND WHY WOULD SOMEONE USE ONE?

Different names for the same technology

You'll hear a variety of terms used for the same general type of technology. Artificial pancreas (AP) or "artificial pancreas system" (APS) is one name. "Looping" is a shorthand name used for "closed looping" (but can also refer to 'open' looping as well). The FDA, among others, like to call them "automated insulin delivery" (AID) systems. Some people talk about "hybrid" vs "fully automated" closed looping. And to differentiate between self-built, do-it-yourself (DIY) systems, you'll see "DIY" prefaced in front of those words to differentiate from commercial types of technology.

To help understand the different names you may encounter, you can see this example visual similar to the one JDRF used years ago to describe the progression in technology:

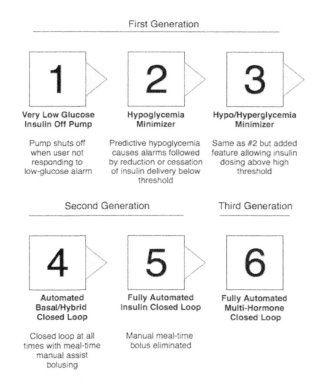

First Generation

1 → **2** → **3** →

Very Low Glucose Insulin Off Pump	Hypoglycemia Minimizer	Hypo/Hyperglycemia Minimizer
Pump shuts off when user not responding to low-glucose alarm	Predictive hypoglycemia causes alarms followed by reduction or cessation of insulin delivery below threshold	Same as #2 but added feature allowing insulin dosing above high threshold

Second Generation — **Third Generation**

4 → **5** → **6**

Automated Basal/Hybrid Closed Loop	Fully Automated Insulin Closed Loop	Fully Automated Multi-Hormone Closed Loop
Closed loop at all times with meal-time manual assist bolusing	Manual meal-time bolus eliminated	

- **Stage 1:** low glucose suspend. When your glucose passes a certain low threshold, insulin is reduced or suspended.

- **Stage 2:** predictive low glucose suspend. When your glucose is predicted to pass a certain low threshold, insulin is reduced or suspended.

- **Stage 3:** hybrid closed loop. When your glucose is predicted to pass a certain low threshold, insulin is reduced or suspended, and when your glucose is predicted to pass a certain 'high' threshold, insulin is increased.

- **Stage 4:** also hybrid closed loop.

- **Stage 5**: fully automated closed loop. No manual mealtime entry required.

- **Stage 6:** fully automated multi-hormone closed loop.

As you can guess, this image was created over a decade ago. (JDRF first started talking about and funding their "Artificial Pancreas Project" in 2006). Now, stage 3 & 4 are essentially the same thing, and are both considered to be standard "hybrid" closed looping, and is the current reality of commercial closed loop systems coming to market in the next several years.

However, would you believe that stage 5, or 'fully automated' closed looping is already a reality for some people in the DIY APS world?

Choose one - what would you give up if you could?

What do you have to do today (related to daily insulin dosing for diabetes) that you'd like to give up if you could? Counting carbs? Bolusing? Or what about outcomes – what if you could give up going low after a meal? Or reduce the amount that you spike?

How many of these 5 things do you think are possible to achieve together?

- No need to bolus
- No need to count carbs
- Medium/high carb meals
- 80%+ time in range
- no hypoglycemia

How many can you manage with your current therapy and tools of choice? How many do you think will be possible with hybrid closed loop systems?

With just pump and CGM, it's possible to get good time in range with well-timed meal boluses, counting carbs, and eating relatively low-carb (or getting lucky/spending a lot of time learning how to time your insulin with regular meals). Even with all that, some people still go low and have hypoglycemia. So, let's call that a 2 (out of 5) that can be achieved simultaneously.

With a first-generation hybrid closed loop system in the DIY community like the original OpenAPS oref0 algorithm (first released in early 2015), it's possible to get good time in range overnight, but in order to achieve that for meal times would still require bolusing and counting carbs. But with the perfect night-time BGs, it's possible to achieve no-hypoglycemia and 80% time in range with medium carb meals (and high-carb meals with Eating Soon mode etc.). So, let's call that a 3 (out of 5).

With some of the advanced features we added to OpenAPS with oref0 (like advanced meal assist or "AMA" as we call it), it became a lot easier to achieve a 3 with less bolusing and less need to precisely count carbs. It also deals better with high-carb meals, and gives the user even more flexibility. So, let's call that a 3.5.

However, in early 2017, when we began discussing how to further improve daily outcomes, we also began to discuss the idea of how to better deal with unannounced meals. This means when someone eats and boluses, but doesn't enter carbs. (Or in some cases: eats, doesn't enter carbs, and doesn't even bolus). How do we design to better help in that situation, all while sticking to our safety principles and dosing safely?

In order to better help in those situations, we designed some new components of the algorithm (including a way to "supermicrobolus" and safely front-shift insulin activity by borrowing from future basals).

With these features enabled, it is possible to achieve a solid 4 out of 5. **And not just a single set of 4, but any 4 of the 5** (except we'd prefer you don't choose hypoglycemia, of course):

- With a low-carb meal, no-hypoglycemia and 80+% time in range is achievable without bolusing or counting carbs.

- With a regular meal, the user can either bolus for it **or** enter a rough carb count / meal announcement and achieve 80% time in range.

- If the user chooses to eat a regular meal and **not** bolus **or** enter a carb count, the BG results won't be as good, but the system will still handle it gracefully and bring BG back down without causing any hypoglycemia or extended hyperglycemia.

That is huge progress, of course. And we think that might be about as good as it's possible to do with current-generation insulin-only pump therapy. To do better, we'd either need an APS that can dose glucagon and be configured for tight targets, or **much** faster insulin. The dual-hormone systems currently in development are targeting an average BG of 140 mg/dL, or an A1c of 6.5, which likely means more than 20% of time spent above 160 mg/dL. And to achieve that, they do require meal announcements of the small/medium/large variety as well.

Fiasp is promising on the faster-insulin front, and has allowed some users to choose completely unannounced and un-bolused meals, but it's probably not fast enough to achieve 80% time in range on a high-carb diet without some sort of meal announcement or boluses. However, 4 out of 5 isn't bad, especially when you get to pick which 4, and can pick differently for every meal. This is what we are achieving with DIY APS, which are essentially second-generation systems - and we hope (and expect that) the same type of flexibility in choices and outcomes will be possible with second-generation commercial systems as well.

How APS works

Whether we're talking DIY or commercial systems, hybrid or fully automated systems, they all essentially work the same in terms of their most basic functionality.

This type of technology makes small adjustments every few minutes to provide more or less insulin with the goal of keeping blood glucose (BG) levels in a predefined target range. It does so with the following components: an insulin pump, a continuous glucose monitor (CGM), and a controller.

In "manual" diabetes mode, *you* as the human are the

controller. You look at information from your pump and CGM, do some mental calculations, and decide what to do. And you do it over and over again, all day, every day.

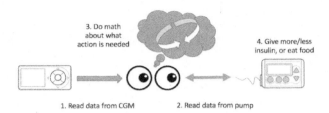

Manual diabetes:

3. Do math about what action is needed

4. Give more/less insulin, or eat food

1. Read data from CGM   2. Read data from pump

5. Do it again.. and again... and again...

@DanaMLewis

In "automated" diabetes, a computer functions as the controller in the middle of the system. It reads from the pump and CGM, does calculations based on your settings, makes predictions about what might happen, and changes insulin dosing in order to change the predicted outcomes to your blood glucose levels.

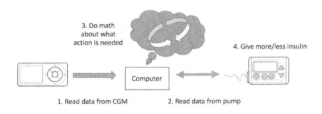

Automated diabetes:

3. Do math about what action is needed

4. Give more/less insulin

Computer

1. Read data from CGM   2. Read data from pump

5. Do it again.. and again... and again...

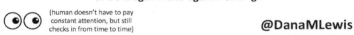

(human doesn't have to pay constant attention, but still checks in from time to time)

@DanaMLewis

A computer is much better suited to be the "controller" than we humans. We humans have lives to live, jobs to work, the need to sleep, etc. As a result, even the most attentive human will sometimes take a break or do something else and not be able to constantly track BG levels. A computer can be told to watch for every new incoming BG data point, every five minutes, and re-calculate and re-adjust accordingly.

Another reason a computer works so well in an APS is that diabetes is complicated and has numerous, incalculable factors that we have to respond to - but can't always count or track. For example, stress and adrenaline and excitement may influence your BG levels, as does activity and exercise. But sometimes they may make your BG rise, and other times your BG will drop. Sometimes it's instantaneous, and sometimes it may happen hours later. It can be hard to predict and adjust for manually. So it's better to wait and see what happens, and make constant adjustments, but we humans don't have the time or patience for that.

Additionally, insulin is not instantaneous. Modern "rapid" acting insulin peak around 60-90 minutes, and have a tail that still influences your body 6-8 hours later. That can be hard to keep track of. Modern pumps' bolus wizards attempt to help with that, but they don't take into account temporary basal rates that may have adjusted your insulin delivery or time spent suspended (because you were swimming or showering). Training the controller to track the insulin activity curves and both the negative and positive impact of more or less insulin delivered compared to your body's normal is a lot easier than us humans doing the task constantly!

In other words, diabetes is hard. It's constant. It's unrelenting. A computer will watch carefully, constantly, and be able to respond more quickly than a human does in most situations to fluctuating blood glucose levels. And if it's unable to respond enough in an extreme situation, it can be designed to alert you to the need for more insulin or carbohydrate intake.

Different closed loop systems will require different levels of interactions from you as a human. Depending on your goals and preferences, that may influence both your choice of what type and brand of system to use, and it also may influence your choices in how you interact with that system over time.

Analogies for understanding the impact of APS on living with type 1 diabetes

A newborn baby

When I try to describe the impact of APS to people who don't have a close knowledge of type 1 diabetes, I first have to start by giving them a better understanding of type 1 diabetes. And not just "the pancreas no longer produces insulin", but an understanding of *living* with type 1 diabetes. This means giving them an analogy for how much diabetes can disrupt and take energy away from normal life activities. It doesn't always, but it can.

The best analogy I've found that resonates with a lot of people is that of a newborn or young baby. Babies need care, feeding, holding, etc. every few hours. It doesn't matter if you are tired and want to sleep: they may wake you up by crying so you can take care of their needs. Sometimes the usual things work to check and solve the problem: you can feed them, and they'll go back to sleep. You can change their diaper, and they'll go back to sleep. Sometimes you're mystified and nothing's working and the baby won't stop crying, so you can't go back to sleep. Even on a "good" night, you're still being woken up. You have sleep deprivation, and you're exhausted.

With type 1 diabetes, it's like a newborn baby that never, ever grows up. In the middle of the night, your blood sugar level may drop. It could be from a number of reasons, such as exercise the day before. Your blood sugar may rise, due to delayed carbohydrate absorption or a late-night dinner. It could be from a hormone surge from dawn phenomenon, or a growth spurt. It could be because your menstrual cycle is approaching. For any number of reasons, your blood sugar could be out of range, and it may wake you up - either from your CGM alarming, or because the symptoms of the high or low wakes you up. You may have to wake up enough to think through what you need to do. It may be a quick fix, or it could involve staying up a while until your BG levels normalize. And there is no cure for type 1 diabetes, so this is the reality from diagnosis onward.

With an APS, it's like having a "night nanny" for diabetes. When your BG starts to rise or drop, the APS will respond and do everything it can to take care of the problem for you. It might still need to wake you up, but instead of several times a week being woken up in the middle of the night - and in some cases multiple times per night - you might experience only having to wake up once a month, or once every six months. The difference can be huge - and that's just talking about the nighttime aspects of living with type 1 diabetes!

Spoon theory

The other analogy that sometimes resonates is that of "spoon theory". It's a concept used in the chronic illness community to help describe how much energy and work it may take to just live regular life while dealing with the chronic illness, and originally coined and described by Christine Miserandino.

Think of it this way: you may have five "spoons" for a typical day. On a good day, it may take one spoonful of energy to do all your diabetes-related task. That may leave you a spoon for going to the gym and working out, a spoon for work, a spoon for playing with your kids, and a spoon to spare for something else. On a day after you were woken up twice overnight to deal with low blood glucose levels, it may take two spoons' worth of energy, leaving you with only three spoons for the rest of your day. If it's a typical day, it might be ok. But what if it's a day where you need two spoons for work, or your kids need more spoons, etc.? It can make it hard to do everything, or even to just function "normally" throughout your typical day.

You could also think of it in monetary terms. What if you had one dollar ($1) to spend every day on things you loved doing? What if diabetes normally "costs" forty cents ($0.40) to do the other activities you loved? If APS could give you back thirty cents ($0.30), what else could you do with that time, energy, and better health?

Why people may choose to use APS

There are numerous reasons why people may choose an artificial pancreas system.

My reason, as I indicated in the preface, is around sleep: I want to be able to sleep safely and with peace of mind. There is nothing better for me than a long (say, 10-12 hours) night of sleep with my blood glucose levels staying within target range all night long. Some people have been able to achieve this on MDI or standalone pumping - I never was able to do this consistently due to my changing activity patterns. I also appreciate the security of having the system, day or night, responding to any fluctuations in BG levels for whatever reasons.

That's not the only reason people choose APS technology. Some people choose it because they can achieve the same goals (A1c) with much less work. Sulka Haro & his family do a great job of articulating this, because they were able to count their manual records of how many treatments they did on a daily basis for their son's type 1 diabetes. Before starting OpenAPS, they made an average of 4.5 manual insulin dosing corrections per day. (Can you imagine the work to chase a young toddler around all day and ask them to eat when they don't want to, or stay still long enough to bolus on their pump?) That number doesn't include routine actions like meal-boluses and carb corrections. After OpenAPS and choosing their preferred features and algorithm adjustments over time? They now do less than an average one manual insulin correction per day. It's a huge reduction in the amount of work they have to do, while achieving the same A1c as before.

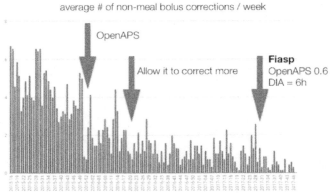

average # of non-meal bolus corrections / week

OpenAPS

Allow it to correct more

Fiasp
OpenAPS 0.6
DIA = 6h

Another story I think is valuable to share is the Wittmer family's story. Jason Wittmer built an OpenAPS rig for his son. Katie Wittmer also happened to work in the school district, so they were able to gain access to the records of the number of times their son had to go to the school nurse. In 4th grade, before OpenAPS, he had to go to the school nurse's office - and leave class and his peers - 420 times in the school year. That's an average of 2-3 visits per day. 354 were "routine" visits for pre-lunch or pre-gym checks. 66 were visits for hypo- or hyperglycemia. Compare that to their 6th grade experience: he only visited the school nurse five times. (Three of the visits were from gym-associated hypoglycemia; two were malfunctions from the CGM or OpenAPS rig where he needed help troubleshooting).

The primary motivation for most people using DIYAPS is

to improve glycemic control, and sometimes the improvements can be dramatic.

Mary Anne Patton describes her experience starting OpenAPS after 38 years living with type 1 diabetes, in her blog, myartificialpancreas.net. She says OpenAPS gave her the tools to see, for the first time, how her extreme insulin sensitivity and blood glucose volatility had led her to develop compensatory behaviors to avoid hypoglycemia, and that these were affecting her glycemic control. She graphed her last 13 years of A1c results, and showed the point at which she started on a DIY APS.

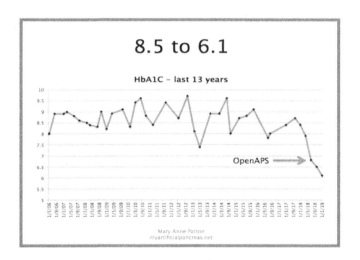

One good overview of peoples' motivations for choosing DIY systems, which is likely to be similar to the reasons people have for choosing commercial systems, comes from a survey done in the DIY community via the OPEN research collaboration, of which I am a part. This is a grant-funded initiative to study the open source diabetes space. The survey was presented at ATTD 2019. Some of the top responses about motivations were around reducing short- and long-term complications of diabetes. I appreciate this survey because it allowed us to differentiate between the choices and responses of individuals (adults) with type 1 diabetes, compared to caregivers' (parents and/or spouses) choices of motivations. For caregivers, their own sleep is usually a key driver of choosing an APS solution.

It may not matter what other people's reasons are, though. Everyone is different: our diabetes may be different. Our lifestyles are different. Our goals, choices, and preferences are different. So at the end of the day, it's a personal decision about whether or not you'd like to use an APS, and which APS you'll choose to use.

2. CHOOSING AN ARTIFICIAL PANCREAS SYSTEM

When choosing an artificial pancreas system, you have a number of choices to make.

1. DIY or commercial?
2. Hybrid, or fully automated (if/when available)?
3. Open, or closed looping?

As discussed in the previous chapter, there's a variety of different types of APS and related systems, which I won't rehash here. I also won't go into details on all of the specific commercial systems. Instead, here are some things to think about to guide your choices.

What matters most to you?

The most important thing to consider is what matters most to you. You may have strong preferences about the manufacturer, type of pump, type of CGM, or even the size, shape, and colors of systems. Other choices can include some of the following.

Physical components

- **CGM**

  Some systems will have only one CGM choice: choose the system, and it comes with the de facto CGM. Others will have options for CGM. Eventually, and ideally, most systems will come with a choice of CGM.

- **Pump body**

  You may strongly prefer the look of one pump over the other. You may want a tubeless option, a small pump, or a pump with a large reservoir. You may want a waterproof pump. You may want an option that is less likely to alarm going through metal detectors. You may care about how the pump is charged, or what batteries it uses. You may care about which sites work with the pump.

- **Controller**

  The controller may be integrated into the pump body. Or, it may be a separate device - this could be a standalone, locked-down controller that cannot be used for anything else. Or, it could be something that can be installed on an Android or iOS phone. You may feel strongly about having to carry "one more thing". Or, you may not trust the security or reliability of your existing mobile device (or the Bluetooth connectivity) to act as the controller for your APS. You may prefer to power and charge the controller separately, or you may find you are better able to keep it running if it's on your primary phone.

Algorithms, features, and flexibility

Most of the first-general commercial systems will focus on the above components. But the algorithm and its capabilities, plus the advanced features and other flexibility of usability choices may (and in my opinion, also should) influence your choice of system.

- **Algorithm**

  You may feel strongly about using a particular algorithm, which you may have used before from a clinical trial, read studies about, or used in a different system. Some algorithms may have different features than others.

  Note: don't focus too much on things like "basal-only" systems vs. "microbolus" systems - those are just different technical terms for how insulin gets delivered, and are often used to distinguish versions within the same family of algorithm. You should also evaluate the algorithm's ability to reach blood glucose targets, time in range targets, etc., which will be covered later.

  If you choose a particular commercial system, and they

have an improved or updated algorithm, how will you get updates or the next version? Will it cost more? What happens if this is inside or outside of your device warranty cycle?

- **Targets**

  Both default, regular targets and temporary targets may matter to you. The regular or default target can make a big difference. The first commercially approved AP system targeted 120 mg/dL, and the only alternative was a temporary activity target of 150 mg/dL. That may be ok with you, or you may want different targets and flexibility.

  In the DIY community, all systems have flexible targets. We use temporary targets to adjust insulin delivery leading into and during/after physical activity. We also use lower than usual targets as a way to adjust insulin delivery prior to a mealtime. Flexibility in targets is very useful for eliminating many every-day spikes and drops, even with a second-generation-capable APS.

- **Data entry**

  If you dislike having to handle your pump or have situations for work or otherwise where you might want to be discreet, consider whether you have to enter carbs and adjust targets on the pump. Or can you use the secondary mobile device, or your own mobile device? This could mean your mobile phone (Android or iOS), or a smartwatch.

- **Remote monitoring, or secondary displays**

  Remote monitoring can be useful for many reasons. (As an adult with diabetes, I still find it useful to have my loved ones be able to remotely monitor as needed.) Will your system of choice have remote monitoring capabilities built-in? If not, does it work with one of the DIY remote monitoring capabilities?

  Remote monitoring can also enable your own "glanceable" displays on your phone or smartwatch of choice. Think about widgets for your phone or your computer, your watch, and other devices such as your car. Will you be able to access your data in real-time and get it to the device you want?

  And, what data will it display? Is it just CGM data? What about knowing if your closed loop is currently automated and working as expected? What about predictions and alerts? What about your net IOB?

- **Calibration**

  You may also want to find out about the management of your APS as it relates to your CGM. For example, does the system stop you from looping (and fall back to manual pumping) if you don't calibrate your CGM per the recommended schedule? How does it warn or alert you to the need to calibrate, or the end of your CGM sensor?

- **Real-world behaviors and interactions**
  How does the system deal with the following real-world situations?
  - If you forget to bolus for a meal (but usually do)
  - If you forget to enter your carbs for a meal (but usually do)
  - If you ate, but threw up (food poisoning, etc.)
  - If you have gastroparesis and have delayed digestion
  - If your pump site has fallen out, and you haven't gotten the insulin delivered that it thinks you have
  - If it's been learning that you're resistant because your pump site is too old, how do you tell it when you've changed your pump site? Does the learning algorithm take that into account, or can you tell it so?
  - What happens when it breaks? How will you get support, or a replacement? How quickly can you get a replacement? What does manual mode look like after you've been on your APS?
  - Will it alert you if you need carbs?
  - Will it alert you if it can't give you more insulin, or if it's been giving you the maximum amount it can give you for a certain period of time?
  - Is this device likely to add to your diabetes burden or

reduce it? Ease of use is important.

Examples for making your choices

One helpful resource for answering some of the above questions about coming-soon commercial devices is Diatribe's list of upcoming US and EU-based artificial pancreas systems, which you can find at https://diatribe.org/artificialpancreas. Not all manufacturers will have released enough data and information about their systems to answer the questions above, but hopefully when a system is released to the commercial market, there will be enough information about the above to help you make an informed choice. If the manufacturers don't release enough information to answer all of the detailed questions, you might need to wait until someone in the community gets their hands on one and writes up a more detailed real-world review.

I'll use some of the examples from the DIY world to show you how answering of the above questions may drive your APS choices.

For starters, you need to know your choices. In the DIY world, that's generally OpenAPS, Loop, and AndroidAPS. At a high level:

- OpenAPS works with older Medtronic pump models, can be used with any CGM, uses a separate micro-controller "rig", and can be used with either Android phones or iPhones.

- Loop has a different algorithm than OpenAPS, also

works with older Medtronic pump models or the "Eros" Omnipod, can be used with most CGMs, uses a separate radio device (such as a RileyLink) to bridge communication to an iOS device, and uses an iOS device (usually an iPhone) as its controller.

- AndroidAPS uses the OpenAPS algorithm, works with DANA*R(S), DANA*I, or Roche Combo or Insight pumps or "Dash" Omnipod, works with most CGMs, and does *not* require a separate radio device or controller because the controller is an Android phone. *(It also works with "Eros" Omnipod or older Medtronic pumps with a radio bridge device.)*

Generally, all the DIY systems are similar hybrid closed loop systems. They're designed to send temporary basal rate commands to the pump. They have hardware and software safety limits for insulin dosing, which you can adjust based on your preferences, and change those over time. You can set and adjust your regular targets in addition to setting temporary targets. If they break, or the controller battery dies, or it fails for any number of reasons, at the end of the temporary basal rate, they fall back to standard pump operation.

Common scenarios might include:

- You have access to an older Medtronic pump, but don't care which phone you use. You can choose between OpenAPS or Loop or AndroidAPS, depending on which algorithm you want to use and whether you want your controller to be on an iOS device or not.

- You only have an iOS device and an older Medtronic pump. Your choices are still between OpenAPS and Loop - both can use an iPhone. It's then a question of whether you like Loop's algorithm and interface (and you'll carry a RileyLink), or OpenAPS's algorithm and using a similar sized rig (to the RileyLink) to be both controller and radio.

- You have a Roche Combo or DANA*R pump, and an iPhone. Until a device driver is written for those pumps and the iPhone, you can either switch primary phones to be an Android device, or choose to buy a small, secondary Android phone to be your controller, and in either case use AndroidAPS.

- You like the OpenAPS algorithm, and have an Android phone. In this case, you can choose between AndroidAPS (if you have or can get a compatible pump), or using OpenAPS (if you have or can get an older Medtronic pump). OpenAPS is rig-based and doesn't require a particular phone type.

Tips for making your choice(s)

Here are some other things you should consider when making choices about your APS:

1. **Picking one kind of technology does NOT lock you into it forever.**

   If you're DIYing now, you can choose a commercial system later. If you start on a commercial system, you can still try a DIY system. Also, you can add on components of DIY systems (such as remote monitoring, or Autotune reports) with a commercial APS.

2. **Don't compare the original iPhone with an iPhone X - compare apples to apples.**

   Let's be blunt: the Dexcom 7plus CGM is a different beast than the Dexcom G4/G5. And the G6 is different from those. Similarly, Medtronic's original "harpoon" sensor is different than their newest sensor tech. The Abbott Navigator is different than their Libre.

   Don't be held up by perceptions of old tech – whether it's CGM, pump bodies, or algorithms. Make sure to check out the new stuff with a somewhat open mind, and truly compare apples to apples. These things in commercial systems should change over time in terms of algorithm capabilities, targets, features, and usability. They certainly have in DIY – we've gotten smaller pancreases, algorithm improvements, all kinds of interoperability integration, etc.

If you're reading a review online about someone's experience with an APS, make sure to pay attention to which version they're using. A lot may have changed since the review was first written.

3. **All systems (DIY and commercial) have pros and cons.**

They also each will have their own learning curves. Some of that learning is generalized, and will translate between systems. But like switching between iPhone to Android or vice versa – your cheese gets moved and there will be learning to do if you switch systems.

4. **Remember, everyone has different preferences and choices – and everyone's diabetes is different.**

Figure out what works well for you, and rock it! And when your life changes or your preferences change for whatever reason, know that you'll have choices then, too. If for now, you don't think you (or your teen, for example) would remember a separate controller or be willing to carry it around with you, an all-in-one system where the controller is embedded within the physical pump might be ideal. If later you decide that remembering to carry something with (or something else on) you is worth the benefits of another system, you may decide to switch systems.

5. **Focus on what outcomes are most important - and apply - to you.**

For you, the ideal outcome may be less work on your diabetes. It could be a different A1c, or an improved Time in Range (TIR) goal. However, while some of the research studies will talk about A1c and TIR and many people will share theirs, remember to also ask about what targets the person has set, how much time they spend closed looping, and how much work it is to use or maintain their system. One metric may be most important to you, but be careful to not use one metric that is not representative of the entire APS experience when making (or sharing) your choices.

3. GETTING STARTED WITH YOUR APS

A helpful mindset to start with

It's very common to feel overwhelmed when considering or trying out new technology. But having an open mind as you get started can help. Here are some tips as you get started:

- **It won't be perfect, or easy, at first.**

  It will take time to adjust to the learning curve of your new APS. If you were on a pump before, you may remember the switch from MDI to pump. It wasn't easy or perfect right away. It took time to adjust your settings. It took time to figure out all the features you could use.

  The same will be true with your APS. You'll start with the basics. You'll likely need to adjust your settings with the new system. It will take some experimentation and getting used to the system helping to "correct" for highs and lows.

In fact, you may find yourself wondering why it gave more or less insulin... and then realize later why it did so. This learning period involves learning to trust the system, and also understanding its limitations. You will likely also learn from asking others about how or why the APS made the dosing decision that it decided was needed.

- **Expect it to get better over time, but expect to have to work in different ways.**
  It will likely take a little more work up front in order to achieve better outcomes, including the benefit of less work over time! You may spend more time at the beginning reviewing reports and adjusting settings. Many people find themselves asking "why am I high" or "why did I end up going low?" Sometimes it's "just diabetes". Other times you can identify where your manual actions may have counteracted the system's attempts to do the most optimal thing.

When you go into automated insulin delivery mode, you have to figure things out again just like you did when you went on a basic pump. You need to be able to figure out what's happening and why it's doing what it's doing, so if you're not happy with what's happening, you can make a change. Why are you running high? Why are you running low? Knowing why it's doing what it's doing is critical for adjusting – either tweaking the closed loop settings, if you can, or adjusting your own behavior. Especially in the first few cycles of new tech, you'll have a lot of learning around "I used to do things like X, but now I need to do them like Y."

- **Knowledge of your diabetes is the most important thing.**

  At the end of the day, even with automated insulin delivery, you're in charge. If something doesn't feel right, you can always stop (or pause) and switch back to manual mode. You should still be prepared to deal with, and treat, hypoglycemia. It will still happen. You may find over time, though, that you can treat low blood sugars with fewer carbs than before, if the automated system has been reducing your insulin delivery as your BG dropped over time. And similarly, you may still need to occasionally manually treat for hyperglycemia, but not as much as you would have before. And always, before taking manual correction, make sure you know how much insulin on board you have!

Switching to automated diabetes mode: autopilot for your diabetes

An artificial pancreas in any form of automated insulin delivery isn't a cure. You still have diabetes. You still need to change your pump site. You still may have to calibrate your CGM sensor. You will still need to change your CGM sensor periodically.

It's very similar to "autopilot" for planes - especially because they still have a pilot. With an APS, you're still around and piloting, even if you have automated help from the technology. You're still in charge of flying the plane.

You can think of one CGM sensor session like a "flight". You don't loop (automate the insulin delivery) when you're not wearing CGM or when you're not getting sensor data, so inserting your CGM sensor is like getting ready in the "pre-flight" stage. Once you have CGM data going, you can "take off" and the system can start calculating and making adjustments. But if your CGM rips out or the session ends as planned, you'll be back in manual mode until a new CGM session is started.

Pick a good time to start

When you run a race, one common piece of advice is not to run a race in new clothes, or with a new type of energy bar, etc. The same goes for getting started with an APS. Don't turn on your APS right before a big presentation at work, the night before your marathon, etc.

Instead, plan to start your first APS session when you have a little bit of time. Why? Well first and foremost… it's exciting! You should enjoy the feeling of switching to automated insulin delivery mode. But also, you'll have questions and run into issues. It will take time to learn what you need to do differently, and to monitor the system. Having a little more time to focus, adjust to the new method of insulin delivery, and changing your behavior will make it less stressful.

What do you need to know before you start?

You'll find me repeating comments about changing your behaviors. Some of your behaviors will change immediately, and more will change over time. Especially as it relates to first treating, and later preventing contributing to, hyper- and hypoglycemia.

As you start, make sure you know:

- What is my BG target? When does it correct differently for hyper- and hypoglycemia? Is it a single target, or a range? How can I adjust the target, if at all? How can I adjust it for a short period of time vs. adjusting my regular target?

- How do I bolus? Do I use the bolus wizard? What happens if I bolus on the pump or in the app? What happens if I don't use the bolus wizard? Do I enter carbs for meals? What happens if I don't enter carbs? What if I forget to enter or bolus for carbs? Should I enter carbs for hypoglycemia?

- How do I know if the system is in automated mode? What do I do if it's not automating insulin delivery? How do I turn it on/off if I need to? How do I know what it's doing?

- What does it know? What is it predicting will likely happen? Will it alert me if I need to take action?

- How can I monitor it on a different display or device? What alarm controls do I have? Are my alarms for CGM glucose levels, or are there also predictive alerts and system status alarms?

- When, and how, can I adjust my settings and preferences, or change which features I use?

Settings adjustments

One of the most frequent things people need to do when starting a closed loop system is adjust their settings. Many people are using settings that reflect the 10-years-ago-reality of their body's insulin needs. Other people have tweaked things over time, and their settings are actually wrong in multiple (partially offsetting) ways, but somehow they're getting ok outcomes. It's hard - for both people with diabetes *and* healthcare providers - to adjust pump settings.

Historically, most people have guessed basal rates, ISF, and carb ratios. Their doctors may use things like the "rule of 1500" or "1800" or body weight. But, that's all a general starting place. Over time, people have to manually tweak these underlying basals and ratios in order to best live life with type 1 diabetes. It's hard to do this manually, and hard to know if you're overcompensating with meal boluses (aka an incorrect carb ratio) for basal, or over-basaling to compensate for meal times or an incorrect ISF.

But this can be the difference between 70% and 90% time in range, and up to a percentage point difference in A1c. After all, an automated insulin delivery system uses your settings as a starting point for its calculations. For someone with reasonably tuned basals and ratios, that works great. But for someone with values that are way off, it means the system can't help them adjust as much as someone with well-tuned values. It'll still help, but it'll be a fraction as powerful as it could be for that person.

We learned quite a lot about this in the early days of OpenAPS. We designed OpenAPS to fall back to whatever values people had in their pumps, because that's what the person/their doctor had decided was best. However, we know some people's settings aren't that great, for a variety of reasons. (Growth, activity changes, hormonal cycles, diet and lifestyle changes – to name a few. Aka, life.) One of the most frequently asked questions was - and still is - about how to achieve better outcomes after the initial improvements from closed looping. And probably 90% of the time it comes down to adjusting the baseline settings.

Autotune

In the DIY world, we ended up creating a tool called "Autotune". Autotune is designed to iteratively adjust basals, ISF, and carb ratio over the course of weeks – based on a longer stretch of data. It draws on a large pool of data, and is therefore able to differentiate whether and how basals and/or ISF need to be adjusted, and also whether carb ratio needs to be changed. For safety, none of these parameters can be tuned beyond 20-30% from the underlying pump values. If someone's autotune keeps recommending the maximum (20% more resistant, or 30% more sensitive) change over time, then it's worth a conversation with their doctor about whether the underlying values need changing on the pump – and the person can take this report in to start the discussion.

Autotune was originally designed for use on OpenAPS rigs

specifically, but the feedback was so positive and the demand was so high that the community worked to build ways to make it possible for anyone to run Autotune, even without an OpenAPS rig. This meant Loop & AndroidAPS users, as well as non-DIY closed loop users, could analyze their data and generate recommendations for how they might change their settings.

Now, it's worth noting, that like the other DIY technologies, this is not an FDA-approved tool. However, it's being used regularly by hundreds of individuals to adjust their settings. So if you either are already tracking CGM data in Nightscout, and are willing to add boluses/temp basals/carbohydrate data for a week, you can set up and run Autotune as well. It doesn't matter which type of pump you have. (There have also been a few MDI users who have chosen to run it).

Manually adjusting settings - common patterns to watch for

If you can't, or don't want to use Autotune, there are still other ways to evaluate your settings. One of the most common issues is that people have their basal rates set too high, and then a low carb ratio or ISF to compensate. If you're closed-looping and seeing lots of insulin reduction overnight, chances are your default basal rates may be too high. Similarly, around mealtime, if the system has to add a lot of insulin, your carb ratio may be too "weak", and those basal rates too high.

Note: It's very important to understand that you should only change ONE thing at a time, and observe the impact for 2-3 days before choosing to change or modify another setting (unless it's obviously a bad change that makes things worse, in which case you should revert immediately to your previous setting). The human tendency is to turn all the knobs and change everything at once, but if you do so, then you may end up with further sub-optimal settings for the future, and find it hard to get back to a known good state.

Hills and valleys, peaks and troughs, up and down

Sometimes people observe "roller coasters" in their BG graph. Remember this is all relative - to different people, BG rising and falling by 20 points may or may not be a big deal (but a 50 point rise or drop might feel like a roller coaster).

First, you should eliminate human behaviors that cause these. Usually, it's things like giving a traditional dose of "fast carbs" (such as 15g+ of sugar, glucose tabs, candy, etc.) that is more than needed for a low or a pending low, unless you have significant levels of insulin on board. Remember the system is reducing insulin, and so you often need way fewer carbs to deal with a low, so you may rise afterward if you do too large of a carb correction. Overcorrections like that generally can't be fixed by changing settings: you have to also change behaviors. Ditto for human-driven drops, e.g. by rage bolusing or otherwise bolusing too much when BG is high.

Human behaviors set aside, if you are still seeing hills and valleys in your BG graphs, consider the following:

- ISF may be off, so you may want to raise ISF to make

corrections less aggressive. Remember, make small changes (say, 2-5 points for mg/dL, and .5 or less for mmol) and observe over 2-3 days.

- If you're seeing highs followed by lows after meals, your carb ratio (CR) may need adjusting. One common mistake is to compensate for rapid post-meal rises with a very aggressive CR, which then causes subsequent low BG. One tool for preventing meal spikes is setting an "eating soon" low temporary target before and/or right after a meal, to get more insulin started earlier, and then allow your APS to reduce insulin once the temp target expires, to help prevent a post-meal low. Similarly, a small manual "eating soon" bolus up to an hour before a meal, or a larger prebolus right before a fast-carbs meal, can help match insulin timing to carb absorption without increasing the total amount of insulin delivered (and subsequently causing a post-meal low).

It can be hard to adjust to the idea that your settings need to be changed. There can be some emotional ties or challenges with how much insulin you have been, or need to be taking. You may also have been told to have a certain percentage of basal compared to bolus insulin. However, many of the old rules and recommendations were developed decades ago, and are no longer relevant guidelines for optimizing settings.

The bottom line is that if you're using an APS, expect to need to change your settings compared to what you were using before.

4. TROUBLESHOOTING YOUR APS

Your APS, like any other piece of technology, will break sometimes. One of the things you've probably become well aware of as a person with diabetes is how things might fail. We people with diabetes (PWDs) are well known for having "emergency backups" for most things. Depending on your APS, you may or may not be able to have an "emergency backup", full APS system ready to go. However, some of the broken components can often be fixed, or troubleshooted, and resolved.

If your system breaks, or you stop looping, you should think through the reasons of why you are not looping. There are three major categories of things that will prevent you from looping:

1. No CGM sensor data

2. Wonky or missing data

3. Communication errors between pieces of a system.

Some of these issues have more obvious fixes. If you don't have a CGM sensor running, you won't be able to automate your insulin delivery. It may be a matter of inserting a new sensor and waiting for the warmup period. However, there may also be issues with the quality of data that prevent you from looping. For example, if your CGM shows an error message (such as "???", Lost Sensor, Weak Signal, etc.), your system cannot loop off of that information. In that scenario, you'll have to decide to wait until data comes back, or decide to switch to a new CGM sensor. Additionally, if your controller cannot read your CGM data for any reason, you won't be able to loop, even if the data and the sensor are "good". This could be because your body is blocking transmission from your sensor and transmitter to the controller, or because the controller is out of range. It could also be caused by the Bluetooth being turned off on your controller. It may also be that the environment around you is very "noisy" and interfering with your Bluetooth connections between your devices.

It's helpful to understand these basic scenarios so you can walk through them for troubleshooting if you are alerted, or discover, that you are no longer successfully in automated insulin delivery mode.

If you've chosen an APS that has the controller inside the

pump, that removes one area of troubleshooting. For non-integrated systems, device troubleshooting includes assessing the connection and data transfer between your CGM and the pump/controller.

If your APS has a separate handhold controller or it's on your phone, you'll need to include investigating the connection between the controller/phone and the pump, as well as the controller/phone and the CGM. You may also need to charge your phone more often than you did before.

Your APS may also be working locally, but your loved ones monitoring it remotely may not be able to see that it's working, or you may not be able to see what it's doing on your secondary displays. In that case, you would be troubleshooting the data flow from your controller (pump, separate device, or on your phone) with your uploader device (often, your phone) for transmitting the information to the cloud. Next, you might look to ensure that your phone/uploader has internet connectivity via cellular service or a Wi-Fi connection. Depending on how you're sharing your data remotely, there are likely other troubleshooting steps specific to your setup, but checking the flow of data from your device to the cloud often resolves many of the most common issues. Fixing these can involve killing and restarting a CGM data app, toggling the Bluetooth on your device(s) on and off or even rebooting the devices if possible.

What happens when real-life diabetes happens?

The hardware (or physical) components are often the

easiest to troubleshoot. However, real-world diabetes can sometimes cause issues, too. For example, what happens when your insulin pump site gets pulled out by a doorknob? What happens when you have been running resistant, realize your pump site is "a little bit old" and decide to change it - how does your APS know that your likely cause of resistance is gone? Additionally, how does the APS know about - and deal with - you taking additional insulin, either as an injection or via another mechanism such as inhalable insulin? What happens if you've bolused, and throw up due to food poisoning? And what happens when you travel, with regards to time zones and jet lag and the changing insulin demands that it causes?

You may not have all the answers, or experience all of these scenarios, when you first get started with an APS. But they certainly happen! So it's worth discussing and exploring how your system can potentially deal with these scenarios.

Here's a handy checklist of real-world diabetes things to ask manufacturers of APS about:

- ☐ How long does it take the APS to resume looping after I've had a compression low, an error code (such as ???) or having missing CGM data?
- ☐ How common is it for the CGM reading to be blocked by the body?
- ☐ How often are people in fully closed looping mode with your system?

☐ If my pump site falls out or isn't working well, how do I tell your system that I haven't actually received the insulin it thinks that I have gotten?

☐ Can I tell the system about other insulin sources, and if so, how?

☐ What happens if I throw up after a meal bolus, and/or don't get to eat the meal I accounted for?

☐ When, and how, should I change the time zone on my device when I'm traveling to a different time zone? How will this affect my APS?

☐ What should I do with my APS when I shower or swim? How does it account for, and handle, missing insulin during that time frame?

It's also important to make sure that you know how to switch between closed loop, and open loop, modes. There may be times where you have a scenario like running a marathon down pat, and would prefer to be in manual mode instead of automated mode. Knowing how to do that up front will reduce a lot of stress and uncertainty when it actually is time for you to switch between modes.

Asking for help

Even armed with all of this knowledge, and years of experience, you may still find yourself in need of help from time to time. You need help troubleshooting your new device, you can't find documentation or answers to your question and the support line for your system is closed, etc. Thankfully, the diabetes community is incredibly helpful, friendly, and supportive! There are dozens (if not hundreds) of channels where you can find help and support: forums such as TuDiabetes or Beyond Type 1, Twitter, Facebook Groups, Reddit, etc.

It's not always clear how to ask for help, though. It can be hard to do so. Having spent the last five years interacting and supporting others in the DIY diabetes community online, we've developed some helpful tips to help people who need to ask for help. When some of this is used to post a question online, it becomes easier - and quicker - for someone else to step up and help you work through your issue or scenario.

When possible, try the following:

1. **Start by explaining your setup.**

   DIY example: "I'm building an Edison/Explorer Board rig for OpenAPS, and am using a Mac computer to flash my Edison."

   Commercial example: "I'm using APS XYZ and am attempting to remotely monitor with Nightscout."

2. **Explain the problem as specifically as you can.**

   DIY example: "I am unable to get my Edison flashed with jubilinux."

Commercial example: "I'm unable to see BG and looping data from APS XYZ in Nightscout."

3. **Explain what step you're stuck on, and in which page/version of the docs.**
   DIY example: "I am following the Mac Edison flashing instructions, and I'm stuck on step 1-4."

   (And if you can, paste a URL to the exact page in the documentation or guide you're looking at. Clarify whether your problem is "it doesn't work" or "I don't know what to do next.")

   Commercial example: "I tried doing Step Z but it did not resolve the problem and BGs are not appearing."

4. **Explain what it's telling you and what you see.**
   Pro tip: Copy/paste the output that the computer is telling you rather than trying to summarize the error message, or share a screenshot.

   DIY example: "I can't get the login prompt, it says "can't find a PTY"".

   Commercial example: "I'm looping just fine on APS XYZ, but the error message in Nightscout is ABC. Here is a screenshot: (image)"

5. **Be patient waiting for a response!**

   There are many people who can chime in and help, but even with thousands of people with diabetes out there, they may not be on your channel of choice at that moment. Don't worry if you don't get a response in minutes. If after a while (say, a few hours) you haven't seen any response, you can comment and try to "bump" your post, or check another channel to try to find help.

   Caution: be careful about posting the same question to multiple channels at the exact same time. It can make it hard to troubleshoot across multiple channels, and it also may convince people that your question is being answered elsewhere.

6. **Be aware of what channel you're in and pros/cons for what type of troubleshooting happens where.**

   My suggestions:

   1. Facebook – best for questions that don't need an immediate fix, or are more experience related questions. Remember you're also at the mercy of Facebook's algorithm for showing a post to a particular group of people, even if someone's a member of the same group. And, it's really hard to do back-and-forth troubleshooting because of the

way Facebook threads posts. However, it IS a lot easier to post a picture in Facebook.

2. Gitter or similar for DIY setups – best for detailed, and hard, troubleshooting scenarios and live back-and-forth conversations. It's hard to do photos on the go from your mobile device, but it's usually better to paste logs and error output messages as text anyway (and there are some formatting tricks you can learn to help make your pasted text more readable, too). Those who are willing to help troubleshoot will generally skim and catch up on the channel when they get back, so you might have a few hours delay and get an answer later, if you still haven't resolved or gotten an answer to your question from the people in channel when you first post.

3. Email groups – best for if no one in the other channels knows the questions, or you have a general discussion starter that isn't time-constrained

7. **Start with the basic setup, and come back and customize later.**

Make sure you walk before you run. The documentation for DIY and guides for commercial setups are designed to support the general use cases. The best practice for either DIY or commercial setups would be starting with the basic features and getting familiar before trying to further tweak and customize things. If you skip steps, it makes it a lot harder to help troubleshoot what you're doing if you're not exactly following the documentation that's worked for dozens of other people.

8. **Pay it forward.**
   Don't be afraid to jump in and help answer questions of things you do know, or steps you successfully got through, even if you're not "done" with your perfecting your APS yet. Paying it forward as you go is an awesome strategy and helps a lot!

When possible, try to avoid the following:

1. **Avoid vague descriptions of what's going on, and using pronouns such as "it".**
   Troubleshooter helpers have no idea which "it" or what "thing" you're referring to, unless you tell them. Nouns are good. Saying "I am doing a thing, and it stopped working/doesn't work" requires someone to play the game of 20 questions to draw out the above level of detail, before they can even start to answer your question of what to do next.

2. **Don't get upset at people.**

Remember, anyone responding to your question is trying to help and donating their time and expertise. That's time away from their families and lives. So even if you get frustrated, try to be polite. If you get upset, you're likely to alienate potential helpers and revert into vagueness ("but it doesn't work!") which further hinders troubleshooting. And, remember, although these tools are **awesome** and make a big difference in your life – a few minutes, or a few hours, or a few days without them will be ok. We'd all prefer not to go without, which is why we try to help each other, but it's ok if there's a gap in use time. You have good baseline diabetes skills to fall back on during this time. If you're feeling overwhelmed, turn off your APS, go back to doing things the way you're comfortable, and come back and troubleshoot further when you're no longer feeling overwhelmed.

3. **Don't go radio silent.**

Report back what you tried and if it worked. One of the benefits of these channels is many people are watching and learning alongside you, and the troubleshooters are also learning, too. Everything from "describing the steps ABC way causes confusion, but saying XYZ seems to be more clear" and even "oh wow, we found a bug, 123 no longer is ideal and we should really do 456." Reporting back what you tried and if it resolved your issue or not is a very simple way to pay it forward and keep the community's knowledge base growing!

Also, once you've solved an issue, consider hitting the "edit" button and putting [SOLVED] or [RESOLVED] at the front of your post, so people know that you no longer actively are needing help on that particular issue.

4. **Don't wait until you're "done" to pay it forward.** You definitely have things to contribute as you go, too! If someone's description was really helpful, consider writing that up in more detail and sharing it again with someone in the future, or add it to some of the community documentation for that particular APS system.

Also, don't hesitate to ask for help if you need it. In the Resources section, I'll list some of the online groups such as the "CGM In The Cloud Off Topic" group on Facebook where just about any question goes! Just remember or refer back to some of the above tips and chances are you'll be able to resolve any issues more quickly.

5. MAINTENANCE MODE: WHEN YOU'RE SUCCESSFULLY LOOPING

When everything goes well and your APS is running, it can feel like you're flying. If you're like me, you may get to the point where you wake up in the mornings and only "remember" to check what your BG levels were overnight after you've worked your way through reading your email and checking your phone. When you feel like your APS is working well for you and everything clicks, it seems like diabetes is on autopilot compared to the old manual way of doing all of that work.

However, there are still some critical diabetes-related behaviors required for closed looping. After all, when flying, even on auto-pilot mode there's still a pilot in the cockpit of the plane. Similarly, you're still in charge of your body, even with an APS on hand.

Some of the basic maintenance behaviors you may be used to if you're a long-time pump or CGM user. However, don't be surprised if even long-time pump and CGM users have behaviors that could (and maybe should) be changed when looping.

Pump site hygiene

For example, the length of time you wear your insulin pump site in your body. You may have a habit of wearing your sites for X days. Some people "do ok" wearing them longer than the sites are designed for. However, with a closed loop, it may show you that "doing ok" in manual mode was really not doing as well as you thought, but it was masked by the noise of all the other chaos of manual diabetes mode. With a closed loop, you may have data to show that your pump sites are effective for 2-3 days rather than 4-5-6-etc. With so much other noise taken care of by an APS, the "weak link" remaining in the system (how insulin is delivered into your body) can become more apparent.

CGM sensor lifetimes and calibration hygiene

Additionally, changing and calibrating your CGM sensors (or validating their calibrations) is also a crucial behavior. Many people choose to "restart" and reuse their CGM sensors for a longer period of time. Some of that is out of necessity due to the cost of the sensors, especially if they are self-funded for CGM sensors and must pay cash out of pocket for them. However, many people who start looping, even if they're self-funded, may find that they no longer want to stretch their sensors as far. The sensor can become less accurate over time. Your diabetes may vary (YDMV), and you do you, but if you're currently in the camp of restarting sensors 3-4 times, I wouldn't be surprised if you slowly cut back on the number of "restarts" you do for each sensor. When a sensor gets to be near the end of its life, it can have periods of missing data (where you can't loop), as well as jumpy data. The jumpy CGM data point can cause your APS to oscillate and sometimes overshoot. At best, it can just be annoying. At worst, false and inaccurate data can cause you to get insulin when you didn't need it - or not get insulin when you did need it.

Remember that your APS is mathematically driven. It takes data in, makes a decision, and sends a command out. If the data in (CGM data in particular) is inaccurate, that therefore influences its calculations, predictions, and decisions.

In most modern APS, you may have a choice of a calibration-free CGM device. It may come factory calibrated. You may want to test and validate your sensors at first to determine if you trust them for automating your insulin delivery uncalibrated. If in doubt, you may want to keep a meter on hand to check your BGs, even with a "calibration-free" CGM. You may also decide the benefits of a more accurate CGM are worth calibrating your CGM periodically.

Monitoring

It's essential to have a monitoring system in place, no matter which APS you choose. You should still have CGM alarms that work (and will wake you up if needed), with hyperglycemia and hypoglycemia settings, regardless of whether you're looping or not. However, ideally your APS will also alert you as to whether you are in automated mode or not. This is important for knowing that you're off "autopilot" and are back in manual diabetes mode.

Body recalibration may occur

Don't be surprised if you find yourself feeling differently after the first few weeks on an APS. I don't just mean more well-rested and awake from all the extra sleep you're likely getting! As you spend more time in range, and less time fluctuating between being high and low, your body will begin recalibrating to this "new normal".

It's common to find that the symptoms you might get for a "really high" BG (whatever that might have been for you) might now occur at "moderate high" BG levels. Similarly, some people with hypoglycemia unawareness may find themselves becoming aware of different levels of hypoglycemia, even if they didn't experience any symptoms before.

This may continue to change over months and years. Think of it as the "boiling frog" analogy, but for your body. When you try to stick a frog in boiling water, it hops out. It's hot! However, if the frog is in normal temperature water and it eventually warms up to boiling, the frog is less likely to notice the change in temperature.

Similarly, when your body (if you have type 1 like I do) began to be less and less able to produce insulin, it didn't happen all in one day (most likely). You gradually over time had less and less insulin, and you may have been accustomed to feeling a little bit "off" or "bad" over time until you reached the tipping point or had specific symptoms that caused you to get diagnosed.

So in reverse, as your BGs spend more time in range, your body will get re-accustomed to spending more time in range, and less time in the extreme ends of the blood glucose level spectrum. You'll also have fewer sharp swings back and forth from the extremes, and so your body will get used to that.

The good news is, you're having better days and overall better outcomes and likely quality of life. But yes, it is common to feel "worse" at different levels and experience symptoms of hypo- and hyperglycemia differently than before. It's not just you!

6. TURBULENCE WHEN LOOPING

To continue using my favorite analogy related to flying and autopilot, it also means we have to talk about turbulence and things that can disrupt you from looping. Like the things that can prevent looping in the first place, there are things that can throw off your looping.

Compression lows

I already mentioned wonky sensor data that may mean either a blip in your looping time, or may prevent your insulin dosing from being automatically adjusted. Again, your sensor life and your calibration practices will likely change with looping. But there are also common issues like "compression lows". This can happen when your sensor is physically compressed by laying on it or leaning up against something. This can reduce the fluid flow around the sensor, causing the sensor to detect that there's less glucose. On your CGM graph it can look like a sharp, drastic fall toward a low BG. It's common for there to be two or three data points with a huge, sudden drop, then maybe missing data. Eventually, the data will likely resume on the same trend line as before the drop started. If your APS requires you to have a certain number of continuously recorded data points from your CGM, recovering from a compression low may mean that you won't be looping for a while. It's helpful to know what to expect, so you know what you can - or can't do - to deal with the situation of wonky CGM data.

Body sensitivity changes

But the other big disturbance, so to speak, is around body sensitivity changes. You know all the ways it can happen: you're getting sick, recovering from getting sick, getting ready for/or are on/or are right after your period, or have an adrenaline spike, or have hormones surging, or have a growth spurt, or just exercised, etc.

This is what makes diabetes oh-so-hard so often. But this is where different closed loop systems can help, and one area in particular you should ask about when picking a system: how does it adjust and adapt to sensitivity changes, and on what time frame?

In the DIY world, we've developed a number of techniques to deal with changes in body sensitivities. In OpenAPS and AndroidAPS, we use a feature called "autosensitivity". It looks back at what was expected to happen compared to what did happen over the most recent 8 and 24 hour time periods. It then calculates whether you're running sensitive or resistant - compared to *your* normal, and creates a ratio as a proxy for how sensitive or resistant you are. That ratio is then used to adjust the calculated insulin needs accordingly. This means it will respond to changes in sensitivity over a short time period automatically, and not require any human intervention to detect changes over those time periods.

For shorter time periods - say, you just started throwing up from food poisoning or norovirus, and you know with 100% certainty that you are suddenly and very differently more sensitive to insulin. In that case, you'd likely want to temporarily use a "profile switch" to change your settings. This is common in AndroidAPS (and eventually might be added to Loop) to enable people to switch their profiles to pre-configured amounts different from their usual basal rates, ISF, and carb ratio. In OpenAPS, and likely with some commercial systems you can accomplish the same thing using a high temporary target. Making precise profile adjustments can be hard to do, though, if you don't know what is happening or why, and how much you need to adjust your settings by. Ideally, your APS will automatically detect and respond to changes, but it may take some time to pick up on those changes. In the meantime, you may want to instruct the system to behave more conservatively until everything settles out.

Growth spurts and hormone-related insulin changes for things like menstrual cycle and different stages of pregnancy also cause changes to insulin needs. One of the DIY tools, Autotune, which we already mentioned in the "Getting Started" chapter, can help you make more frequent changes and stay ahead of the settings changes you may need for those scenarios. Hopefully there will be more tools, and guidelines for different scenarios, in the future as APS becomes more broadly tested over a larger and more diverse population of people living with diabetes.

There are also issues related to food digestion: things like acute onset sickness like food poisoning, norovirus, or the flu can all cause you to throw up, or things like gastroparesis can cause intermittently slowed and unpredictable digestion. This can be problematic if your algorithm isn't designed to have a dynamic carbohydrate absorption model. If you frequently experience these issues, it's worth exploring to see if a different algorithm has a different way of dealing with dynamic absorption of food that gives you different outcomes. The difference between a dynamic and a static model (which assumes all carbs are equal and will hit at the predicted time, no matter what) can be significant.

Exercise and changing activity levels

Exercise and activity can be the other major source of turbulence of looping. There are a few reasons why this is the case. First, remember that insulin does not act instantaneously. The insulin can be hitting peak activity at the time of your activity, which can contribute to a major low during your exercise (or after). Additionally, exercise can increase your insulin sensitivity both during and also hours after your exercise. On the flip side, not all exercise will send you low. Certain types of activities can actually drive your blood glucose up - especially things like sprinting or other activities where you are pushing yourself past your current comfortable level of fitness. All of this combined makes exercising with diabetes hard. And an APS makes it easier, but there are still challenges.

Hopefully, your APS will be like the DIY systems and allow the setting of different temporary targets. These are important not only for during and after your activity, but also before your activity commences. You don't want to go into exercise with a lot of insulin on board. Think about the timing - if you eat lunch and bolus, then go for a walk an hour later, that insulin is peaking at the time of your walk. Additionally, the insulin can have an increased effect due to your extra activity from your muscles. Finally, exercise can also delay and slow digestion, so even if you have a meal on board, this can all contribute to a low (and a rebound later when digestion of the meal resumes).

An example of good intentions but misunderstanding the timing

I have a pretty good example of how it took me several years to finally understand how much the timing of everything matters for exercise. In 2013, I decided to run a marathon. I wasn't a runner before, so I was actually starting from step zero in terms of learning how to run: increasingly my running distances, and figuring out how all to do this with diabetes. (And this was before I had built OpenAPS, so I was figuring it out the hard way!)

I worried about going low during the runs. I generally would set a low temporary basal rate to reduce insulin during the run, and try to run before dinner instead of after (to reduce the likelihood of running with a lot of active insulin in my body). I would also eat some kind of snack for energy as well as making sure I didn't go low. I would also carry a bottle of Gatorade to drink along the way in case my blood sugar dipped. And here's what happened:

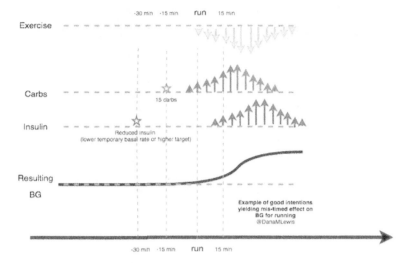

Per the visualization, the carbs would hit in about 15 minutes. If I reduced insulin at the time of the run, it would drive my blood sugar up as well, over a longer time frame (after around 45+ minutes as the lack of insulin really started to kick in and previous basal impact tailed off). The combination of these usually meant that I would rise toward the middle or end of my short and medium runs, and end up high. In longer runs, I would go higher, then low – and sip Gatorade, and have some roller coaster after that.

In the past year (beginning in 2018), I started running more again. This time, I had OpenAPS and was armed with a lot more knowledge and visibility into what was going on. I realized that if I was running in the afternoon or evening, the most important thing to do was to set a higher temporary target (e.g. "activity mode") well before I went out for a run. This could be an hour or two hours before I ran, depending on how much IOB I had at the time. This helped OpenAPS know to reduce insulin accordingly, cutting down on the pool of super-active IOB I had at the start of my run. I also stopped proactively taking carbs (unless I wasn't able to get below about 0.75U of IOB before I started), and just used carbs during the run if I started dropping. It made a big difference, and I was able to run distances around half marathons without any lows and without needing many supplemental carbs to ward off lows, either.

Post-exercise sensitivity matters, too

There are numerous ways that you've likely learned in manual mode to deal with post-exercise sensitivity. Thankfully, an APS can do most of the heavy lifting and dealing with the hard part of not knowing when or how much sensitivity will be impacted. When comparing and choosing APS and talking about people's experiences, if you're someone who does a lot of activity, don't forget to ask people about how well their system deals with post-exercise sensitivity changes. There are certain things you can do manually to alert your system to impending sensitivity changes - such as setting a longer, higher temporary target in our system, but you'll want to pick a system that allows you to do that, and a system that can respond to shorter-term sensitivity fluctuations and not one that takes days to "learn" there's been a change.

Disconnecting from your pump

Disconnecting from your pump for any reason - during a shower, for a swim, etc. - can be a major source of turbulence in your BG levels, even with an APS level. Why? Well, if your BG starts rising, you don't have the pump on so the APS can't provide you with more insulin. It's back to manual mode, where you have to decide to do a correction bolus, reconnect your pump and enable your APS, or otherwise deal with the situation. The other reason it can be challenging is again due to the timing of insulin.

If you're off of your pump for a two hour swim and your BG starts rising, you may decide to reconnect your pump and do a manual correction bolus. However, you've missed two hours of basal insulin. Your bolus will take ~60+ minutes to start hitting peak activity - so you will likely see your BG rise for another hour before the insulin takes effect. It doesn't matter how good your APS is: it's only as fast as correcting for rising BGs as the insulin can take effect.

As a result, you may decide to reconnect periodically and do some small boluses to substitute for basal insulin, in order to keep a little bit of insulin going in your body. You may decide to switch APS's (or pumps) temporarily to one that is waterproof, if yours is not. And some people even choose to swap back to MDI (or at least injected basal insulin) for long pool/beach related vacations.

Sickness or surgery

As you live real life with your APS, you're still human - and if you're like me, your autoimmune system is still a tad overreactive and you may find yourself getting sick from time to time. Not diabetes sick (e.g. not feeling well because of a high or low), but "normal people" sick with the flu or another virus.

Again, it's helpful to know what your system can do. Ideally, your APS will roll with whatever life throws at it.

I've certainly thrown a lot at mine!

In my experience, OpenAPS has successfully handled the following:

- Receiving norovirus from my nephew, and spending three days of not eating at all - but not having a single hypoglycemic/low BG reading (and also no hyperglycemia, or highs)
- Getting the flu and following it with weeks of bronchitis and having excessive insulin resistance and reduced activity
- Falling off a mountain in a foreign country and breaking my ankle in three places, then getting home and breaking a bone in my other foot a week later
- Jet lag from traveling 12 hours' worth of time zones away and dealing with sleep deprivation from missing several nights' of sleep due to red-eye flights

... just to name a few of the most extreme!

When I say successfully, I don't just mean the outcomes (same time in range as if I was healthy), but I also mean the amount of work it required to obtain those outcomes. When I fell and broke my ankle, I was incredibly stressed and in the most pain I'd ever been in my life. I was concerned about having broken bones, I was being winched off a mountain and evacuated in a helicopter to a hospital in a foreign country - by myself, and I wouldn't see Scott (my husband) until he safely hiked out of the trail the following day. I had very little extra energy - and pretty much no extra brain cells - for dealing with diabetes. I had to take zero extra actions with OpenAPS during that entire time period, and weeks later into my recovery. It didn't matter that I stopped moving (and maybe got 10 steps a day, just crutching to and from a bathroom) and stopped eating, or ate more here and there. It didn't matter that I was suddenly eating three times the amount of protein that my body was used to - OpenAPS was able to respond, no matter why. Even when I caught a cold from my nephew, and also had my menstrual cycle at the same time, while dealing with everything else... I didn't have to do any extra work diabetes-wise. It's a huge difference to how things would be if I was having to handle everything in manual mode.

We've also had stories from other APS early adopters in the community, too, around sickness and also surgery. People have had brain surgery, spine surgery, hand surgery, emergency surgeries, and more with APS running before, during, and after their surgeries. Not all surgeons and anesthesiologists are ready to have patients looping during surgery - but several are open to it, so if you find yourself needing to have surgery, it's worth discussing with your medical team. There may not be formal protocols in place, yet, but you can agree upon a protocol including what targets your APS should be using before, during and after surgery, as well as what to do if the system fails, and how the nursing team and others will interact with you and your diabetes differently as a result.

Remember, as always, that your APS is not a cure. You still may have hypo- or hyperglycemia when sick and dealing with things like broken bones, surgery, or recovery. However, your APS should be able to help carry some of the weight of dealing with and responding to fluctuating glucose levels. And the more time you spend in range, the easier it will be for your body to do the rest of its necessary healing.

7. PREPARING FOR YOUR NEXT LOOPING "SESSION"

Unfortunately, it's not always possible to loop exactly 100% of the time. The chief reason for this is that you at some point will need to change your CGM sensor (or it'll fall out and you have to replace it). Remember, no sensor data means no looping. Just like you'll want to plan how you will start on the closed loop, you'll want to plan for how to cycle off and then back on again. Depending on your system, there may be things you can do to smooth things out and limit the downtime of your looping sessions.

"Pre-soak" your CGM sensor if possible

One of the things I do to get better first day results from my closed loop is to pre-soak a CGM sensor to skip the first day jumpy numbers. It makes a big difference for the first hours back on a "new" looping session because it's actually the second 'day' of the sensor, and it's settled in somewhat.

Normally, you'd expect to see a person with one CGM sensor

on their body, like this:

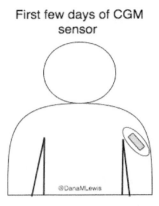

However, 12-24 hours before I expect my sensor to end (or I plan to end the sensor, if it's been restarted already) I insert my next sensor into my body. To protect the sensor (you don't want the sensor filament itself to get torn off or lost in your body), I plop an old ("dead" battery) transmitter on it. If you don't have an old/dead transmitter, you could try taping over it – the goal is just to protect the sensor filament from ripping. Some people also do fine without covering it - YDMV as usual.

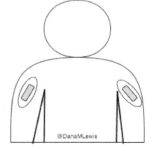

The next day, when my sensor session ends:

- I take the "live" transmitter off the old sensor, and remove the old sensor from my body. I hit "stop sensor" on my receiver, if it hasn't already stopped itself.

- I gently remove the "dead"/old transmitter from 'new' sensor.

- I then stick the "live" transmitter onto the new sensor.

- I hit "start sensor" on my receiver.

After old sensor ends

Switch "live" transmitter to "soaked" (new) sensor, and start your new sensor session.

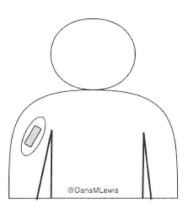

@DanaMLewis

The outcome (for me) has always been significantly improved "first day" BG readings from the sensor. This works great when you can plan ahead and your outfits (don't judge, sometimes you have important outfits like a wedding dress to plan around) and skin real estate support two sites on your body for 24 hours or so.

This doesn't work if you rip a sensor out by accident, so in those scenarios I go ahead and put a new sensor on, put the 'live' transmitter on, and hit 'start' to get through the 2 hour calibration period as soon as possible to get back to having live data. (All the while knowing that the first day is going to be more "meh" than it would be otherwise.)

Depending on your system (both APS and your CGM and your CGM software of choice), you may be able to "restart" or "renew" your sensors without a warmup time period. Some commercial sensors will have a longer life, and/or you may not want to (or be able) to restart them. However, "soaking" your next one has always helped, and never hurt, and may be a good strategy to add to your toolkit to minimize downtime from looping.

Planning for your CGM and looping downtime

Even if you can't pre-soak your CGM sensor you can do some other general planning ahead – like making sure your looping session doesn't end in the middle of a big meal that's being digested, or overnight. Those are the times when you'll want to be looping the most.

I aim to avoid the following situations:

- Pay attention to when my CGM sensor "ends", and sometimes restart it *earlier* than it's supposed to die, so the CGM "restart" time period isn't during a meal, exercise, or overnight

- Try not to eat a meal, and definitely not a large carb-filled meal, during the time when my CGM is warming up. This is for two reasons:

  1. I don't have visibility into what's going on after the meal.

2. My APS can't help out since I don't have data,
so I'm in manual mode and without visibility.

I also try to check when my sensor is inserted and figure out what exactly 7 (or 10 or 14, depending on which sensor) days ahead will be. Where will I be? What will I be doing? If I'm at home and not traveling, and it's during the day or evening, it's less of a big deal. If my sensor start time will come at a time where I'm supposed to be on an airplane, I'll set a calendar reminder for a time before (often the night or day before) to remind me to change or restart my sensor so I have a working CGM and a working APS during my travel. Similarly, I check for what time zone I'm going to be in for the future. If I'd normally be home, but it's 3am in the country I'll be visiting next week, I do the calculations and figure out the time where it will be the least hassle in the middle of my trip to restart or change my sensor. You may be like me if you're a frequent traveler and especially across many time zones and decide that sometimes it's worth a little less use out of a particular sensor to trade off from having to deal with the sensor and changing or restarting it during a busy trip.

Learning from your looping session

Just like learning to fly, where you take a lot of training flights and review how the flight went, you'll want to think about how things went and what you might change behavior-wise for your next looping session. Some of the things that may change over time as you learn more about your tech of choice:

- Timing of meal announcement or boluses

- Precision (if needed, or otherwise lack thereof) around carb counting
- Using things like "eating soon" mode to optimize meal-time insulin effectiveness and reduce post-meal spikes (see more about this in the next chapter)
- Using different activity patterns and targets to get ideal outcomes around exercise

Tweaking underlying settings (if you can)

You'll probably spend more time at the start of your looping journey reviewing your settings and figuring out how things went each time, plus what you might want to change. It's not so different to life overall with diabetes - we're constant tinkerers, experimenters, and scientists. Our bodies and lifestyles are always changing, so we are constantly needing to evaluate what worked, what might have changed, and how we need to respond accordingly. Again, while we have new tech to help, this also throws in new variables for us to experiment with. To help prevent feeling overwhelmed, consider picking one new thing to experiment with each time. Then you can evaluate how it went, decide to continue with the change (or adjust it further), or change back and try something else different.

8. TIPS AND TRICKS FOR REAL LIFE WITH AN APS

One of the most important things I've learned along the way both has to do with APS directly, because it enabled me to learn and understand it, but also applies to *all* individuals with type 1 diabetes, regardless of how they get their insulin injected or delivered. Namely, this is the important of understanding and tracking the timing of insulin.

What we learned several years ago related to carbohydrates and insulin activity timing

One of the most common strategies for trying to better match insulin timing with meals and food-related activity is the "pre-bolus". The definition varies, but when people say "pre-bolus" they usually mean taking some or all of your necessary meal insulin prior to the meal. That could be a recommended 15 minutes prior, or up to an hour prior. This recommendation evolved because we know it takes a while (60+ minutes) for insulin to peak, whereas food will impact BG levels within about 15 minutes. Such pre-boluses do help somewhat in preventing large spikes in BG immediately after meals, but in my experience an 80-point BG rise (from 80 mg/dL to 160 mg/dL, for example) is still common for meals consumed "on an empty stomach" with little or no extra insulin on board (IOB) prior to the pre-bolus. Pre-bolusing can contribute to dangerously low BG (hypoglycemia) if a meal is delayed or if you end up eating fewer carbs than expected. But we've learned a few things in the last years because of our experiences watching the data as we tested first DIYPS and then OpenAPS that has enabled us to develop another strategy for minimizing post-meal spikes.

Here's the detailed explanation of what we learned. If you'd like a shorter and visual explanation, skip to the next section.

- When carbohydrates are consumed, as part of a meal or snack, or to correct a low-blood-glucose (BG) situation, it causes BG to rise, but that rise is both delayed and gradual. In developing DIYPS' model, we discovered that for n=1, there is a delay of approximately 15 minutes between carb consumption and when BG starts to rise as displayed on a typical CGM.

- In addition, we discovered that the rate at which BG rises after carb consumption is fairly constant, both across food types and over time. For n=1, we observed that carbohydrates are digested and absorbed at a rate of approximately 30g/hour (0.5g/minute), and that this rate is relatively constant beginning after the initial 15-minute lag, and lasting until the last of the carbs are absorbed (up to 4 hours later, in the case of a large 120-carb meal).

- We also observed that, for real-world meals, glycemic index (GI) doesn't matter much for carb absorption rate. Our initial testing was performed on high-GI foods used to correct low BG (juice and Mountain Dew) and a milkshake consumed without corrective insulin while participating in an unrelated clinical trial (to try to detect any endogenous insulin production, which was not present). However, in subsequent real-world use of DIYPS, we've observed the same for almost all meal types. It seems that for meals containing at least some sugar, starch, or other highly accessible form of carbohydrates, the body seems to begin digesting and absorbing the most accessible carbs immediately, and is able to break down low-glycemic-index carbohydrates by the time the higher-GI foods are absorbed.

- We also observed that the level of insulin activity at the start of a meal matters a great deal in determining whether BG rises significantly as the meal carbs are absorbed by the body. This actually matters more than the starting level of BG (e.g. having active insulin matters more than you being 80 mg/dL compared to 140 mg/dL). It's not IOB, but insulin activity that matters. We learned this by studying the differences in post-meal BG rises from empty-stomach meals, and meals where there was some insulin activity happening over the past few hours (from BG corrections or a prior meal period).

- Why is this the case? Our theory is that the liver needs insulin when the carbs first hit. When carbohydrates are initially absorbed by the small intestine, they are directed into the portal vein and pass through the liver before reaching the rest of the body's circulatory system. The liver is designed to absorb any excess glucose out of the blood at that point, storing it for later release. The mechanism by which the liver does so is dependent on two factors: the presence of higher glucose levels in the portal vein than in general circulation (indicative of ongoing carb absorption), and the presence of sufficient active insulin. If enough insulin is fully active, the liver can absorb ingested carbs just as fast as they can be absorbed from the intestine. If not, then the glucose passes through the liver into general circulation, and cannot be subsequently absorbed by this mechanism, but must be absorbed later by peripheral tissues once insulin levels get high enough.

- Therefore, a 15 minute pre-bolus isn't enough for getting the insulin fully active in time. Even fast-acting insulin does not reach peak activity for 60-90 minutes after injection, since it must be absorbed through subcutaneous tissue into the bloodstream. This means that if no insulin is on board from previous boluses, the pre-bolus insulin doesn't really kick in for 30 minutes or more after the start of the meal. In the time it takes pre-bolus insulin to kick in, the body might absorb 15-20g of carbohydrates, resulting in a 60-80 mg/dL rise in BG.

- To adjust for this, we needed to find a way to provide insulin even sooner than a typical pre-bolus. But how would you do that safely, without causing low BGs before or after the meal? The best way we've found to do this is to do a tiny and early pre-bolus about an hour prior to a meal. We calculate the size of the early pre-bolus based on the current BG, by determining how much insulin we can safely add and still stay above 80 mg/dL for 1-2 hours. In our case, that means assuming that up to 75% of the insulin activity will occur before the meal carbs kick in. So for a BG of 110 mg/dL an hour prior to the meal, and a correction ratio of 40 mg/dL per unit of insulin, it would be safe to bolus 1 unit of insulin. That 1 U then ramps up to peak activity right at mealtime, and largely prevents any substantial rise in BG immediately after the meal.

- Your mealtime bolus then needs to be adjusted to take into account the IOB. You also don't want to bolus for more carbs than your body can absorb before that insulin hits. For example, a large meal with 90g of carbohydrates would take ~3 hours to absorb, but insulin activity often peaks after 60-90 minutes. If you have a large meal, you might decide to bolus at mealtime for only the first 30g of carbs initially (minus any prebolus), since those will be absorbed over the first 60 minutes. If the meal totals 60g of carbs, you will then want to bolus for the next 30g of carbs over the next hour, possibly via a continual delayed ("square wave") bolus, or by doing one or more manual bolus(es) after the meal is over. Or at least - that's what you would do in manual mode. With your APS, you should be able to do your first bolus, enter your carbs, and let the system take care of the rest.

How to do "eating soon" mode

With an APS, you have an even easier way to do "eating soon" and increase your pre-meal insulin activity. All you need to do is set a lower than usual target for your APS, and it will adjust your insulin accordingly. For many people who run a typical 100 mg/dL "usual" target, they may set an 80 mg/dL target for 60 minutes prior to eating. Even thirty minutes ahead of time can help. Remember, it's not about the amount of insulin - any insulin activity peaking will help reduce a post meal rise. Additionally, if you've been running on the lower end of your range for several hours, this will make an even bigger difference and blunt the likely spike that will happen when you eat carbs and they hit a bloodstream that has not had insulin active for a long time.

If you're not yet on an APS, you can still take advantage of this strategy:

1. If you know you're going to eat sometime in the next hour, manually calculate a correction bolus with a target BG of 80, assuming only ¾ of the insulin you give will take effect by the time you begin to eat. (Example – if your correction ratio is 1:40, and you are currently 110 mg/dL, that means you would use 30 (¾ * 40) to calculate that you

need to give yourself 1U of insulin.) You can give this an
hour, 45 minutes, or 30 minutes prior to the meal –
whatever you make work is better than not doing it!

2. Eat your meal and bolus normally, but use your IOB as
part of your meal calculation so you don't forget about
that insulin you already have going. (It's best if your pump
or APS tracks IOB and you can use a bolus calculator
feature, but if you take injections, keep in mind about the
insulin you've already given for the meal – just subtract
that amount (1U in above example) from what you'd
otherwise inject for the meal.)

Note: if you use eating soon mode, you might want to delay
the last unit or two of your meal insulin until after you see
BGs rise, since sometimes you need less total insulin for
the meal if you get insulin active early. This is especially
true for people who haven't tested their settings in years,
and are in manual mode. Often, we PWDs may
overcompensate with more insulin than we need because
it's not timed correctly compared to the carb absorption
rate. Be careful as you experiment with adjusting your
bolusing strategies and improving your peak insulin activity
time.

Here's a concrete example of manual-mode "eating soon":
- 5pm – You're planning to eat around 5:30 or 6pm. Your

BG is 110 and your correction ratio is 1:40. Setting your correction target to 80 and applying the ¾ ratio, that means you take 1U of insulin.

- 6pm – You sit down to eat. Looking at your meal, you see 45 carbs and decide, with a carb ratio of 1:10, that you would take 4.5 units for the meal. Keeping in mind your earlier bolus of 1U, you end up taking 3.5 units for the meal. (4.5U total – 1U prebolus = 3.5 more units needed to cover the meal, see above note about considering delaying a unit or two of that bolus until you see your BGs impacted by carbs).

You should have less of a spike from your carbs kicking in 15 minutes after you eat. It won't always completely eliminate a spike (you can still be wrong on your carb count, etc.), but it will provide a flattening effect and reduce the spike that otherwise would have occurred.

And here's a visual of what often happens:

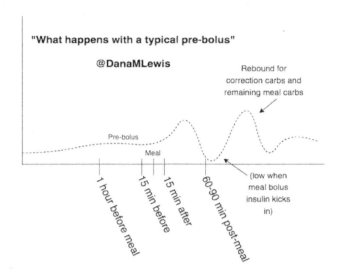

And a visual of ideally what happens with an "eating soon" mode, manually or via a target on your APS:

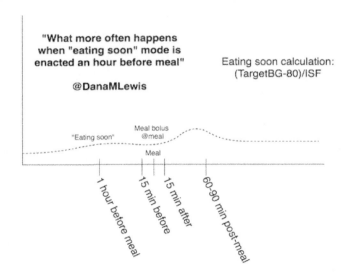

Again, APS users will find it easier to change their target in advance of the meal. If your system is interoperable, you can use things like Google Calendar and IFTTT to adjust your targets ahead of time - including planning an "eating soon" target at different times during the work or school week when you may be more likely to forget otherwise. For example, some families set up a Google Calendar so they can pre-plan target adjustments for the entire weeks' worth of gym class and lunch times. If your system does not allow pre-planned target changes, or temporary target changes, you can still achieve a similar outcome by doing the manual version of "eating soon" to optimize your insulin activity timing relative to your meals.

Changing your pump sites more effectively

In addition to CGM sensors, pump sites are the other "weak link" in your APS. They can get ripped out, they can stop working, and sometimes even on insertion they just don't appear to work... or it takes hours before it seems like the insulin takes effect. It can be incredibly frustrating.

Similarly to "soaking" new CGM sensors, I've developed a practice and changed how I change my pump sites, whenever possible.

What I used to do (i.e. for 12+ years):
- Pull out pump site
- Take shower
- Put in new pump site
- If the pump site didn't work, spend all night high, or the

next hours high while I debated whether it was just "slow" or if I needed a second new site. Ugh.

What I decided to start doing and have done ever since (unless a site gets pulled out by accident):

- On the day that I decide to change my pump site, I do not take my "old" pump site out before my shower.
- After my shower, I leave in the old pump site and put the new pump site on. Which means I am wearing TWO pump sites.
- I put the tubing on the new site etc. as expected. But because I have the old site on, if I start to see BGs creep up an hour or two later, I can do one of two things:
    1. Swap the tubing back to old site, give a bolus or a prime on the old site, then switch tubing back to new site. (I do this if I think the new site is working but seems "slow")
    2. Swap the tubing back to old site, remove the new site, and then insert a second "new" site (or wait until the next morning to do so when I feel like it)
- Otherwise, if BGs are fine, I pull the "old" site out once I confirm the new site is good to go.

The other reason why you should consider keeping the old site on for a while is if you've recently given a bolus or otherwise had a lot of insulin go into the site. Sometimes, if you remove your pump site, you'll see insulin spill out. This can occur even if the site wasn't "occluded". So you actually didn't "get" some of that insulin, which can lead to a high within a few hours, and you'll be playing catch up from the time of the inserted new site and waiting for the new site's insulin activity to kick in, and then playing catch up from the missed insulin that spilled out of the old site. I don't seem to experience that problem anymore when I leave the "old" site on for a few hours after I insert the "new"/next site.

To me, it's worth keeping the old site on for a few (or even ~12) hours. I know many people may not like the idea of "wearing two sites". But it's not wearing two sites for 3 days. And if you find yourself having a lot of post-site-change highs — that's why and when I switched over to this approach.

Traveling with your APS

Have pancreas, will travel!

Just like an insulin pump, an APS can and does travel well. But one of the common questions the DIY and early adopter of commercial APS communities have seen is: what do I do when I travel? What about airport security? What about time zones and jet lag?

Dealing with airport security

A list of diabetes gear you're probably packing for your trip:

- BG meter
- Test strips
- Lancet(s)
- Pump sites

- Reservoirs
- CGM sensors
- CGM receiver
- Tape for sites/sensors
- Syringes as back up
- Anti-nausea meds
- Depending on the length of your trip, backup pump/transmitter/meter/receiver/etc.
- Snacks
- Pump
- APS (if it's a separate rig or controller)
- Insulin
- Extra insulin
- Juice for lows
- Spare batteries

Out of that list, here are the only things I would pull out of your bag when you send it through the x-ray at security.

- Insulin/extra insulin*
- Juice for lows**

Everything else (yes, including your CGM receiver; yes, including your pancreas rigs/APS device) can stay in your bag and go through the x-ray.

*If you have a single bottle of insulin, it's under the liquid (3oz) limits, so you don't technically need to pull it out.

But if you are carrying numerous bottles/pens/etc., if you have them separately bagged and can pull out separately, I would do so in order to reduce the risk of them flagging your bag for needing additional screening.

** Yes, you have a medical need for liquid and can take juice through security. HOWEVER, I *highly* recommend having this in a baggie and pulled out of your bag so it is separate. They'll often pick that up, examine it, and if you say "medical liquid for diabetes", it's fine. Sometimes you'll get pulled for a pat down, but not always. And, this usually prevents them from having to dig through your bags to find the juice and go through all your things. (Which is annoying, not to mention time consuming).

My second "HOWEVER" related to juice: I've stopped carrying juice for lows when I air travel. Yes, it only takes an extra couple of minutes or whatever for them to check things out, but I'd rather not have any hassle if I can avoid it. I instead have switched to Starbursts, Skittles, and similar. (They're super fast acting for me, and actually make it easier to do a small 4g correction vs having to bust open an entire 15g juice box that can't really be saved for later.) I have those in my pocket or easily accessible in an outer pocket of the bag that will go under my seat on the plane. You can of course still carry juice, but think about if that's really worth the hassle/effort and if there's an alternative (glucose tabs, small wrapped candies, etc.) that might be easier for treating lows when traveling. YDMV, of course.

What about insulin pumps? Should or do you take it off?

- It depends on which system you wear. My (Open)APS includes an insulin pump that does not alarm in 99% of metal detectors because it's not made with lots of metal. I also have TSA Precheck, which means 95% of the time when traveling in the U.S. I am only asked to go through a metal detector. So right before I walk up to security, I take my pump that's usually clipped to an outer pants pocket and clip it inside my waist band and underneath my shirt. If it doesn't alarm, then I proceed like a usual traveler to get my bags and be on my way. This is also the case for most building metal detectors. However, if you have a metal-cased pump, you may want to proactively ask for a pat-down if you know it's going to alarm every time.

- If I am randomly selected by the metal detector to instead go through the body scanner:

  ○ If you wear your pump into the body scanner, the system will likely flag it, and agents will likely want to do a pat-down anyway.

  ○ The radiation dosage from a properly functioning backscatter x-ray is tiny: lower than the background radiation you're exposed to every 2 minutes of your life, or every 12 seconds on a plane. There are no guarantees that the body scanners will always be functioning properly and won't break your pump, and a pretty high likelihood that if you go through the scanner you'll still need a pat-down as well. So if you have a super special limited edition rare pump that does a special thing (like those that enable you to DIY closed loop), as I do, it may make you decide that just a pat down is better than a scan plus pat-down, since if it DOES break due to a malfunctioning scanner, TSA sure isn't going to pay to fix it/get you a new one, and a new one wouldn't allow you to DIY closed loop anyway. If you have a commercial APS, you should ask the manufacturer what their recommendations are for body scanners.

o So, if I get randomly selected, I stop right there and say "opt out". Say it to whoever is pointing you over to the body scanner, they'll possibly read you a script to confirm you want to opt out, and just keep saying "yes, I opt out" and "that's fine" to the "but then you have to have a pat down!". They'll order up a same-gender TSA agent who will come get you, escort you around the body scanners, and you'll get your pat down. The usual applies – if you want, you can ask for a private area for your pat down. I usually don't care, but if you do, make sure you keep an eye on your bags and ask for those to come with you so they're not left out in the open for anyone to accidentally take. (They're usually pretty good about that, though.)

- o For the pat down, they'll ask you about sensitive areas/medical devices. This is the time to point out your pump: tell them (pat the area) where it's connected, and pat/point out your CGM sensor if you have one. They'll be extra careful then to not accidentally catch their hands on those areas.

- o At the end, they'll go swab their gloves, then come back and ask you to pat/touch your pump and then let them swab your hands.

- If you don't have Precheck, the above will likely happen every time. So if you're an opt-out-of-body-scanner-type and travel more than 2 times a year... Precheck is probably worth the money if you can afford it. (And think about getting Global Entry, which comes with Precheck included, and also gets you expedited return to the country after traveling abroad).

- If you have a metal-cased pump (or any other pump, and just want this instead of the metal detector or the body scanner), you can ask for a hand inspection of your pump/APS. Different manufacturers say different things about whether x-ray and body scanners are ok/not ok, so check with them and also go with your gut about what you'd like to do with your pump. Keep in mind that the radiation your carry-on luggage gets from the hand-luggage x-ray is many times higher than what your body gets from a backscatter x-ray, so if you're concerned about x-ray radiation damaging your pump, it should not be sent through the scanner with your carry-on luggage.

What about a doctor's note?

I have never carried a doctor's note, and have not had an issue in the 14+ years I've been flying with diabetes – including in dozen of international airports. YDMV, and if you'd feel more comfortable with one, you can get one from your doctor. But for what it's worth, I don't travel with one. I've never had an issue in any country in the world explaining even my DIY-APS components, insulin pump, or CGM.

What about international airports?

The only thing to know about international airports is they have similar guidelines about liquids, so plan to also pull out your juice and toiletries from your bag. Same rules apply for keeping rigs, supplies, etc. in your bag otherwise. I've never had an issue based on pancreas rigs internationally, either. They're small computers and batteries, so both TSA and international security are used to seeing those come through in the x-ray.

Time zones and jet lag

If you're changing time zones when you travel, you have a few options. If you are traveling briefly, or only across a couple of time zones, and would not normally feel the need to adjust the timing of your basals, then you may not want to bother adjusting your devices' time zones. But, if you would like to adjust to the new time zone (perhaps for a longer trip or a move), you can adjust your APS's clock. I recommend planning to do this when you have some extra time for troubleshooting, in case you have issues. It may be confusing if you have to change your CGM separately from your APS, or if your CGM automatically updates to match your phone but your APS does not change its time. Or, it may not matter to you at all - especially if you typically have a relatively flat basal schedule throughout the day and don't see much variation in insulin needs.

More importantly, it's worth noting that your body only changes about an hour or so of time zone a day, so even if you go abroad, there's not a rush to change time zones/the time on your APS - you can wait until 2-3 days into your trip to make the swap. Even if you're jumping ahead 8 or 12 hours of time zones, it will take your body a while to catch up. The changes from being off-shifted from your typical underlying basal pattern will be minor; the bigger changes that the APS will be handling will be the jet lag, sleep deprivation, activity change, and likely food changes from your travel.

Don't forget your emergency backups!

Regardless of the risk from x-ray or body scanner, stuff happens. Murphy's law says it will happen when you travel. Remember to read up in advance and know what your options are for taking or getting a replacement APS on your trip (if possible, and if something breaks that you can't resolve), and have enough supplies to fall back to standard pumping or MDI if necessary.

9. SUCCESS STORIES

At this point, you've likely seen or heard several success stories. Mine, as it related to sleep and dealing with everything my life has thrown at my diabetes. Sulka's and his family's reduction in the work it takes to manage their son's diabetes. Jason's son's reduction in school nurse visits. Mary Anne's dramatic reduction in A1c.

Tim Street also has a compelling way of talking about the benefits of APS. He describes the habits of diabetes, having lived with it for 30 years, and those becoming the "habits of a lifetime". He then describes the evolution of the DIY APS community features:

"We no longer have to do everything to the nth degree, and that's as astonishing as it is gratifying. [...] It's not a cure but it's the next best thing."

In other words, diabetes is so much less work, monitoring, tracking, and everything else involved. This can be incredibly beneficial, and especially for individuals with diabetes who are children or teens.

One teen's father has shared his son's experience and data openly with the DIY community. It's almost astonishing to read - his son is eating a typical teen diet of 200+ grams of carbohydrates per day. His son doesn't want to do anything diabetes related. He doesn't carb count or announce meals. He doesn't bolus. And yet he's achieving 72+% TIR and a 6.2 A1c. He spends very little time doing *anything* diabetes related. This is only possible because he's using APS technology (OpenAPS) and fast-acting insulin (Fiasp): if he didn't have access to an APS, he would either have far worse outcomes, or would have to dramatically change his lifestyle.

Katie DiSimone, a parent of a teen girl with diabetes, has also blogged about the differences before/after choosing to use an APS:

> "Before DIY closed looping, school mornings were such a cluster @#$%. We had huge basal set from 5am-8am plus an extra (always a guess) bolus when she left the house to help control the school morning nerves. And then, this year, she has PE second period... oh but wait... not always second period because it might be a block day schedule. You parents know what I'm talking about... always having to stay on my toes about what day of the week it is and make sure the bolus/basal program is the right one. We regularly battled 220s in the morning using that system. Plus interrupted her school day with about 5 text messages to try to get things right. Then we got on

Loop and OpenAPS… so much better. […] We were pretty happy with this system because we no longer needed to text her, she wasn't overdosing, and our basal switching around was no longer necessary. Win-win-win. […] I don't interrupt with a text message asking what it was. I don't intervene."

Mary Anne Patton also describes her experience in her blog:

"For me, OpenAPS has been a self-correcting system in that it's given me enough of a feeling of control (not just BG control), that I've had the confidence, the breathing space, and finally, the tools, to make further changes to keep my blood sugars in range *even more* of the time, by adjusting my settings and modifying some of my diabetes behaviors.

Before OpenAPS my data looked like a complete scramble. Now I can see **patterns**. And it is such a relief that finally, it isn't just up to me".

This stuff matters.

Diabetes is SO much more than the math – it's the countless seconds that add up and subtract from our focus on school/work/life. And diabetes is taking away this time not just from a person with diabetes, but from our parents/spouses/siblings/children/loved ones. It's a burden, it's stressful… and everything we can do matters for improving quality of life. It brings me to tears every time someone posts about these types of transformative experiences, because it's yet another reminder that this type of technology makes a real difference in the real lives of real people. It doesn't matter if it's DIY or commercial - it works, it makes a difference, and it matters for so many people. It enables people to recapture hours upon hours of lost and disrupted sleep and hours upon hours spent focusing on work or life without distraction or worry.

Justin Walker, another person who's lived with diabetes for 32 years, believes that using an APS has increased his life expectancy. He also estimates that using an APS has given him back a full hour of time every day for the rest of his life.

But it's not just highly motivated individuals with diabetes who succeed with APS technology. One public example is Cameron Chunn. He has shared that before using a closed loop (he ended up choosing to use OpenAPS), he wasn't caring about his diabetes, even when he began to notice some related complications. It wasn't until he had children that he decided to do something more than the bare minimum to keep himself alive.

"Suddenly my life was more than my own, and I had a responsibility to this new life that I had created. I made the decision to take care of myself. I found a new endocrinologist and switched to a pump and a CGM. I managed to lower my A1c from 10.2% to 7.7%. However, it was tons of work and I was constantly watching the

CGM trying to correct highs and figure out how to not have highs, etc. It wasn't great. I then found OpenAPS, and it changed my life. I didn't suffer lows much anymore, and even if I screwed up I knew I'd return to normal without having to fight to do so. My A1c's are now regularly in the 5.7-6.2% range.

I still have bad days (weeks...) where sickness or something else causes my blood sugar to be bad and I can't really control that – but I've gotten to a place where I understand that can't really be helped and you are just going to have a few bad days sometimes.

I'm back to not caring about diabetes. Except now I'm not killing myself in the process.

I'd never tell anyone that it's problem free, or that any of the APS tech is perfect, but the minor hassles of the day to day are miniscule compared to all the mental strain of trying to be your own pancreas. It's 100% worth it, and I'd never go back."

Remember this: your diabetes may (and will) vary (aka, YDMV). Your lifestyle, the phase of life you're in, your priorities, your body and health, and your choices will ALL be different than mine and anyone else's. That's not bad in any way: that's just the way it is. The behaviors I choose and the work I'm willing to do (or not do) to achieve **my** goals (and what my goals are), will be different than what you choose for yours. So what looks like success to me may not look like success to you – and that's fine! What's most important is finding out what success is for you and seeing if APS can help you achieve it. It may, or may not be, things like A1c.

When you ask someone else who's looping (e.g. using a closed loop/APS system) what their A1c is, is that context-free number what you really want to know? Or do you really want to know how well they're doing incorporating the technology into their lifestyle? Are you trying to figure out what you might achieve if you choose APS technology, or what's possible? A1c is often used as a proxy for a variety of things, but it leaves out so many metrics of success that may be equally – or even more – important to someone. That's why I encourage people not to try to compare themselves, or compare others, because it's definitely not going to be equal even with the same, single metric like A1c. It's also important to keep this in mind when reviewing research about APS technology. You need to know what target the system was targeting, what settings they were using, what behaviors they were using, how much and how they were monitoring and intervening with the system, their level of activity or inactivity, and how other behaviors might vary and influence the system.

10. HCPS AND APS

What healthcare providers (HCPs) should know about APS

It is hard to define what HCPs need to know about APS, because they need to know what patients know about APS, too. So if you are a HCP reading this chapter, I hope you'll also take a look at the rest of the book, too. APS has tremendous benefits for patients, ranging from achieving improved clinical outcomes to reducing the burden of managing diabetes and improving quality of life. APS also has benefits for providers, too. It may take away some of the difficulty of helping patients achieve their ideal outcomes, and make the remaining work easier and allow you to focus more on the more fulfilling task of helping your patients make fully informed tradeoffs in their particular situation. But I also recognize that most HCPs have not yet been trained with APS – it still isn't something that is taught in medical school. We are learning together as we go – the early adopters and HCPs – to figure out how best to use APS in real life and clinical care.

It may seem scary for HCPs, especially when patients are leading the way with this new technology. But it's helpful to remember that patient innovation is not new. The patient community leading the way demanding increasing access to new technology is not new. This is even more true in the diabetes field. Do you remember hearing about the advent of at-home blood glucose testing, back in the 1970s? Patients led the way, demanding the ability to test their BG at home. At the time, clinicians were very concerned about patients' decision making abilities and the ability to handle the additional information it provided them.

Does that sound familiar? The same arguments were made about continuous glucose monitoring, and whether patients should be "blinded" (prevent from seeing in real-time) their own data. The same arguments were made about dosing insulin from CGM. The same arguments still appear today around flash glucose monitoring. The same arguments happened when insulin pumps were invented.

It's no surprise therefore that the same concerns are now front and center with regards to artificial pancreas technology and related systems.

"Dear optimist, pessimist, and realist:

*While you were arguing about artificial pancreas technologies…
we've been using it. For years.*

*Sincerely,
The do-it-yourself diabetes community"*

Healthcare technology is well-known for being behind technology in other sectors. And do you know what unfortunately lags further behind that? Policy, education, and tools to help healthcare providers (HCPs) understand how to use, support, and otherwise deal with the technology. I expect that many HCPs might remain unfamiliar or uncomfortable with most APS technology - DIY or commercial - for many years to come. Fortunately, there are outliers! Some HCPs use APS themselves, have been trained on it, are adopting & encouraging adoption and promoting access. Some HCPs are reaching out to learn more from non-traditional resources like this book. But the average experience will be more likely that patients will have to ask for APS, or a different kind of APS than the sole option that might be recommended, and likely end up educating their HCP about other options along the way.

I know that this might sound pessimistic. It's not to scare you off, or offend any HCP who reads this. But, both for DIY or commercial APS, and similar to patients having to ask (and demand) for access to CGM, it's going to take a lot of effort from patients and the community to get to the point where it becomes the new standard of care. I think the patient community therefore have an ongoing, important role to play that doesn't end when more commercial APS are approved to the market. "Approved" doesn't mean accessible, let alone affordable, for patients. And HCPs' attitudes towards this technology are also going to play a role - but hopefully one of increasing access rather than adding additional barriers.

Thankfully, diabetes organizations are stepping up and beginning to release position statements to encourage and emphasize that patients have the right to choose their technology.

Diabetes Australia released the first position statement in late 2018, emphasizing patient choice. JDRF UK followed in February 2019 with a similar position statement, and many others are in the works as well. While there are still cultural questions that remain about liability for physicians, there is a growing awareness and acceptance that patient choice is paramount. As it should be.

We still need HCPs

We still need HCPs. Point blank. APS won't take that way, and it doesn't risk the job of HCPs. In fact, we know there's a shortage of trained endocrinologists and other diabetes-related care providers. If you're a HCP, APS will change the way you work, and what you have to do - but I see this as a good thing. HCPs will be able to work "to the top of your license" and take care of the hardest problems that technology has not yet addressed.

However, companies will need to do a better job with what tools and reports they provide - for both patients, and providers. We need to design carefully the data that is provided to us patients in real-time, as well as for retrospective review. The same goes for HCP reports and the ability to analyze data retrospectively to help spot bigger picture trends and problems that they may spot. Right now, I think HCPs have a hard job to do without these reports and tools. APS should theoretically also reduce the burden on the healthcare team - but hasn't yet. We need it to get there and reduce the cognitive burden on HCPs to match the reduction on workload and cognitive burden that it provides to patients.

What I wish HCPs would know about APS

Sometimes, I see HCPs hear about APS and have a knee-jerk reaction that it must be risky. When they have that reaction, it seems like they forget how risky manual diabetes is for everyone on insulin-dependent diabetes. And the same thing for whether a technology or type of APS is regulated or not. Yes, a regulated or "approved" version of technology means it has been vetted by a regulatory body and approved for general use. But that doesn't mean it's perfect. Again, it's not a cure for type 1 diabetes. It still requires some work on behalf of the person living with it and to figure out how to make it work for them.

I wish HCPs who work with patients with diabetes knew the following:

- When a patient chooses to use a particular technology, it's for a good reason. And, it's worth finding out *why* a patient has made this choice. Especially in the case of a DIY APS. Yes, DIY tech is off-label. But that's ok – it just means it's off label: it doesn't prevent you from listening to why patients are using it and what we think it's doing for us, and it doesn't prevent you from asking questions, learning more, or still advising patients 1:1 about their choices. There is a growing body of position statements to back you up in supporting your patients.

- Patients often dread talking to HCPs about their choices, because they're afraid. They're afraid you'll refuse to listen to us, to discuss it, or that you'll fire us as patients. Please don't make us switch providers by refusing to discuss it or listen to it, just because it's new/different/you don't understand it. *(By the way: we don't expect you to understand all possible technology! You can't be experts on everything, but that doesn't mean shunning what you don't know.)*

- You get to take advantage of the opportunity when someone brings something new into the office – it's probably the first of many times you'll see it, and the first patient is often on the bleeding edge and deeply engaged and understands what they're using, and open to sharing what they've learned to help you, so you can also help other patients!

- You also get to take advantage of the DIY community. It's open, not just for patients to use, but for companies, and for CDEs and other HCPs as well. There are dozens if not hundreds of active people on Twitter, Facebook, blogs, forums, and more who are happy to answer questions and help give perspective and insight into why/how/what things are. In many cases, we're begging HCPs to be involved and connect with the community.

- Don't forget – many of the DIY tools provide data and insight that currently don't exist in any traditional and/or commercially and/or FDA-approved tool. Take autotune for example – there's no FDA-approved tool to help patients tune basal rates, ISF, and carb ratio for people with pumps. And the ability of tools like Nightscout reports to show data from a patient's disparate devices is also incredibly helpful for healthcare providers and educators to use to help patients. These tools for the most part don't exist as regulated tools or software. They may need to be reviewed carefully, and taken with a grain of salt, but that doesn't mean they should be categorically ignored and rejected.

- When asked for advice they would give to fellow HCP's, one HCP emphasized to me that there is likely a network of HCPs supporting this already in your area. And if there's not one, create one! It allows HCPs to learn from one another (in addition to learning from patients). If you can't find any HCPs in your area, look online to the active community of HCPs. Many happen to have type 1 diabetes and are using this technology personally as well as have patients who have chosen to use it.

In summary, for HCPs:

- Please support your patients & their choices.
- Embrace DIY as a learning opportunity for you.
- Connect with the DIY community for help.
- There are a lot of new, exciting tools for you and patients!

New ways of doing things means new methods of evaluation are needed

APS is a new model of doing things in type 1 diabetes. That also means we need to develop new models of evaluating things. Some of the methods developed for "evaluating" patient settings decades ago no longer match these older models. For example, some HCPs strongly believe that there should be a specific, fixed ratio of insulin delivered as basal vs bolus on a daily basis. However, there are a few flaws in this methodology.

Say you think there should be a 50% split between basal and bolus insulin. That means someone should get about 20 units of basal insulin, and 20 units of bolus insulin, if their average total daily dosage (TDD) is 40U. However, that is a simplified rule that conflates three different variables. The body needs a certain amount of insulin throughout the day: that's basal insulin. If the blood sugar is elevated for some reason (leaving out food for a minute), such as stress, exercise, sickness, hormones, etc. - then it needs to be corrected with the "correction factor" or insulin sensitivity factor (ISF). Finally, the third ratio is for food: carbohydrate or "carb" ratio, for how much one unit of insulin will cover how many grams of carbohydrates. If someone eats more carbohydrates one day, they will need more insulin... and you shouldn't decrease the body's baseline insulin needs (e.g. basal) to balance that ratio. The ratio therefore gets distorted.

Trying to force the ratio even from the beginning of putting someone on an insulin pump ends up causing a lot of issues for people with diabetes and their eating habits. They may try to contort what and how they eat in order to match their insulin to the "ratio", rather than what their body actually needs (as baseline and for the food consumed). There is a growing body of evidence around eating disorders related to, and caused by, living with type 1 diabetes. Having a wrong, forced ratio applied to "how much insulin we should be taking" can cause irreparable damage mentally and physically. Plain and simple, it's wrong. Your body needs how much insulin it needs. You also need to take enough insulin for what you eat. What a "healthy" diet for the individual is, is another topic of discussion. But for the most part, "how much insulin" should not be determining the diet. That's backwards.

Then when someone goes on APS, it's common that the HCP who believes in a fixed ratio (such as 50:50) still demands the same output of basal and bolus amounts. But that doesn't make sense, even if you believe the ratio works for manual pumping. The artificial pancreas or automated insulin delivery system is designed to dose insulin in response and in prediction of out of range BGs. It doesn't matter if it's called bolus or basal. It's insulin delivered in response to the BGs. Discussing the ratio of basal to bolus also doesn't work depending on the APS, which might "borrow" from basal in order to "bolus" (or "microbolus") more up front, achieving flatter BG levels. Each APS works a little differently, and defines insulin delivery in different terms. But focusing on the ratio of basal vs. bolus insulin delivery is a distraction from analyzing the outcomes of what someone is achieving: we should instead be looking at BG variability or post-meal excursions, and properly reviewing and adjusting the factors that influence those outcomes.

And one final point specific to APS and measurement: this technology is going to solve a lot of problems and frustrations for patients and improve outcomes. But, it may mean that patients will shift the prioritization of other quality of life factors like ease of use over older, traditionally learned diabetes behaviors. This means things like precise carb counting may go by the wayside in favor of general meal size estimations, because with the new technology both yield similar outcomes. Being aware of this will be important for when HCPs are working with patients: knowing what the patterns of behaviors are and knowing where a patient has shifted their choices will be helpful for identifying what behaviors can be adapted to yield different outcomes. Behaviors, like settings, are something that can be tweaked to adjust the outcomes of living with APS.

What patients should know about taking or talking APS with HCPs

If you are interested in APS, make sure to ask your HCP about it, even if they don't bring it up. Some HCPs won't bring it up unless they feel that their patients are "savvy" enough (whether that's tech savvy, or APS savvy, or some mystical other type of savvy is unclear) to warrant mentioning it. But you don't have to be "savvy" or already educated. If you're interested in the idea of APS, it's absolutely worth discussing with your healthcare team. This pattern of what and when HCPs choose to bring up APS as an option may mirror some of the concerns HCPs originally had around pump adoption and use (and even blood glucose meters themselves, back in the day).

Make sure to advocate for yourself

Depending on where you live in the world, you may be able to access and acquire (or build) your own APS, without much input required from your HCP. In other places, you may need a prescription signed off on by your endocrinologist for the full APS, or components of your APS (such as particular pump supplies and sensors that work with your system of choice).

And in any case, you'll need to decide when and how you talk to your HCP about APS, if you do it on your own. There are a few approaches people take:

- Build their own APS, run it for a while, then bring it up in the next appointment when they have data and results to share from it. Usually, HCPs can see the evidence of what's working well, and say that even if they can't endorse or recommend it because it's off-label (and DIY), they can acknowledge that what the person is doing seems to be working well for them.

- Bring the choices of APS to the HCP, and discuss the options with the HCP, getting input about the choice and decision of whether or not to use a particular APS. In a few cases, HCPs have been very unhappy with patients doing this, to the point where a patient may end up choosing to switch HCPs (if at all possible) to one that is not so upset about a patient choosing or trying APS. Others, thankfully the majority, will have a reasonable discussion - if they have enough information - about the pros/cons of choosing a system. Others may need to seek or be provided information before they can have such a discussion.

Remember to share your resources with your HCP, too

There are some great resources created in the diabetes community. The ones written for patients can often also be great introductory material for HCPs who want to learn more about APS in general, or a particular (especially if it's DIY) type of APS. There are also often HCP-specific guides written to provide a clinician with information they need to know about the basics and how to support patients going on a particular system. For example, we have created a "Clinician's Guide to OpenAPS" to have a single link/single page explanation of the system basics, how it works, what the algorithm does, and how HCPs might help patients fine-tune their settings.

For HCPs who are looking for more materials, we'd love to see more from HCPs, by HCPs, for other HCPs! There are several peer-reviewed papers in the literature addressing the HCP audience, but it's the tip of the iceberg of what's needed. There's a lot of room for more studies, more papers, more online guides, and more tools and tutorials to support your fellow HCPs as you figure out how your work will change with APS. (And if I can be of assistance as you create more material, please do reach out. I'm always happy to review, or spread the word about, any new resource!)

11. RESEARCH ON APS

There's a growing body of research on APS, especially in the last few years. This includes academic algorithms and systems, commercially developed systems, as well as open source-designed systems.

One easy way to get an overview of the APS studies at a high level is to look at a "meta-analysis" of the APS studies. A meta-analysis is a review of data from a number of independent studies of the same subject, in order to determine the overall trend. One recent meta-analysis done in 2017 (*Tsapas et. al, BMJ*) , for example, reviewed 40 studies that involved more than a thousand participants. 35 of the studies were for single-hormone APS; 9 studies looked at a dual-hormone system. The conclusion of the meta-analysis was that time in normal glucose range increased significantly with APS use, both overnight as well as overall. It also reduced time spent low, and usually also decreased time spent high. The study also noted some limitations of current APS research: most individual trials involved small sample sizes and short follow-up duration.

The open source or "DIY" systems also have a growing body of research. There are four categories of studies that have been done or are in progress: self-reported; retrospective; observational; and prospective, randomized control studies.

For example, the first study done on DIY systems is the 2016 OpenAPS Outcomes Study. 18 of the first 40 "loopers" self-reported their outcomes using OpenAPS. As in the meta-analysis above, time in range increased, A1c decreased, and other improvements were seen. However, this is self-reported data so this is considered to be a lower level body of evidence.

To address the criticisms, another study was presented in 2018 as a follow up. Although again the number of individuals studied was small - in this case due to the stringent criteria for inclusion - the outcomes were similar. This time the study was retrospective, based on data collected by individuals before and after they closed the loop. There have been additional retrospective studies on open source automated insulin delivery systems, such as *Melmer et al* (2019) and *Wu et al* (2020). *Melmer et al* found similar findings to the previous retrospective analyses, while *Wu et al* found that open source automated insulin delivery use was associated with significant improvements in glucose management and quality of life among adults with T1D.

In 2018, there were other studies done that are "observational", and done by academic and medical researchers outside the community. Researchers in Italy studied 30 individuals using DIY systems. Researchers in Korea evaluated data from 20 children using DIY systems. These, too, showed similar improvements in time in range, with reductions in A1c, time spent low, and time spent high.

Prospective studies have also been done, using DIY technology. Users of AndroidAPS (the DIY system that uses the OpenAPS algorithm in an Android phone application, connected to a Bluetooth-capable pump) were enrolled during a ski camp to compare the outcomes against a predictive low-glucose management (PLGM) system. This wasn't quite an apples to apples study: the PLGM system only tries to prevent hypoglycemia, whereas AndroidAPS will attempt to correct both hypo- and hyperglycemia. And, the numbers were small: 10 AndroidAPS users and 12 PLGM users. However, this study *(Petruzelkova et al)* was notable because it concluded that AndroidAPS was a safe and effective alternative to a commercially available PLGM.

The same researcher recently presented a study at ATTD (a European scientific conference focused on diabetes technology), and subsequently published the study *(Toffanin et al,* 2019) analyzing both a retrospective group of Android APS users (n=34) as well as preliminary results of in-silico testing. Again, the results of real-world use match the in-silico testing to find time in range increasing, time spent low and high decreasing, etc.

And what about prospective, randomized control trials of

DIY technology? Well, those are coming, too, with data expected from the CREATE trial (see *Burnside et al* for the trial's protocol) in 2022.

I'll keep updating this section as more notable studies come out!

Accessing research

If you're interested in a particular system you're considering, the results from the big studies are usually available at a high level, and sometimes in full detail via abstracts or posters from scientific conferences. You can also usually find them easily via a search engine.

However, sometimes journals are "paywalled", meaning it asks you to pay for a certain article to get access to read it. Sometimes there may be a previous version posted as a poster, or written up in a subsequent meta-analysis. But one little-known method for accessing research? Emailing the author directly! Usually, the copyright agreement for a journal submission allows personal use of the article on a researcher's own website (as long as it's for non-commercial use). Not everyone posts their work on their websites - but every researcher I've ever emailed has been willing to email back a copy of their article! So if you see research that you want to read, contact the author and ask for a copy of their research.

You can also ask your fellow community members for help. Some individuals work at universities or otherwise have access to journal memberships and can help you access a copy of the research article.

Future research ideas

Most of the time our data is looked at in real-time, then forgotten about. But this data often has powerful insights. We can learn from what we're doing as individuals in the real-world, answering questions that have not been addressed by research before, like: How does insulin sensitivity change before, during, and after each menstrual cycle? How often should one adjust settings during pregnancy with type 1 diabetes? Can you detect growth spurts from your diabetes data? The list goes on and on. And the insights gathered from this data can fuel new tools, better APS technologies, and a better understanding overall of aspects of type 1 diabetes that previously has been obscured by noise.

If you'd like to contribute to research, one easy way to do it is to donate your diabetes data. You can donate to a couple of big repositories. If you use Nightscout, you can donate to the Nightscout Data Commons on Open Humans. This enables your data (which is anonymized during the upload process) to be used for various research projects. If you're a DIY closed loop user, you can also donate to the OpenAPS Data Commons. Several studies, like the DIY studies discussed above, have been performed with this data. You'll be directly powering new research projects when you donate your data! There are also places like the Tidepool Big Data Donation Project where you can donate your data.

CONCLUSION

Artificial pancreas technology is here, and it's here to stay. We still have work to do, though. We need to make it available, accessible, *and* affordable to every person with diabetes who wants it. We have to make sure that this tech is flexible enough for people to use in the real world and to achieve the best possible outcomes. We also need to make sure that it's not burdensome for everyday use, and that it works for people who are recently diagnosed with diabetes as well as those with a deeper, longer background of living with diabetes. There are tradeoffs that individuals should be able to make, choosing between their behaviors and the number and type of interactions they have with such a system. And we should have interoperability, so someone can choose the best algorithm, CGM, pump body, and controller type for them.

We also should remember that not everyone will want, or

choose, this type of technology. That's absolutely fine, too. It's about having choices for everyone, which includes the choice to not use APS (or pump, etc.). But, there are things we have learned in our pursuit of improving and developing APS that can apply to help improve technologies available to people without APS. There are management techniques and tricks that can improve life for anyone with diabetes, even if they're not using a CGM. Even if they're on MDI. We need to apply the lessons learned for everyone with diabetes.

We also need to recognize that people with diabetes themselves are the experts in APS. We're the ones using these systems every day and night, and living real lives that are messy and gloriously full of edge cases that a typical medical device designer doesn't think of - or is talked out of designing for, due to the lack of business case. We need to change the system around how these devices and systems are designed so that our feedback as patients is not only listened to, but incorporated into a much quicker design cycle for improving the next version and iteration.

APS technology has incredible benefits for a person with diabetes, their loved ones and friends, and even their HCP. But it requires change. Change for the person managing diabetes, to figure out how they might need to do things differently, and how to troubleshoot new technology. Change by payers/insurers for covering and reimbursing for these systems. Change for the healthcare provider to learn how to evaluate this new technology differently (including how to conceptualize changes to diabetes therapy), and changing what they need do to help support their patients - even if they disagree with their patient's choice of what is right, or best, for them.

***

I remember over seven years ago when we announced that we had figured out how to close the loop. I remember the feeling when we announced OpenAPS and stated that we thought it should be possible for anyone to do APS if they wanted to. I remember the pushback of people saying - it works for you, but what about everyone else? We still get pushback today, telling us what we shouldn't have done. And what we shouldn't do now.

But I remember thinking that if it helped one other person sleep safely at night… it would be worth the amount of work it would take to open source it. Even if we didn't know how well it would work for other people, we had a feeling it might work for some people. And that for even a few people who it might work for, it was worth doing. Would DIY end up working for everyone, or being something that everyone would want to do? Maybe not, and definitely not. We wouldn't necessarily change the world for everyone by open sourcing an APS, but doing so could help change the world for someone else, and we thought that was (and still is) worth doing. After all, the ripple effect may help ultimately change the world for everyone else in ways we couldn't predict or expect at the time.

That's what APS is. It's not a cure. It's a ripple effect. It will affect and influence the life of someone with diabetes in ways they never could have imagined. You may have your own goal or idea of why you want an APS. It might be because it'd be safer, or let you get better sleep. It might be so that you can go back to work and your kid can go to school by themselves. It may be a safer or more easily managed and hopefully healthier pregnancy. It could be to help potentially reduce long-term complications that we can't predict or control.

And I bet you'll be surprised at what else it affects. It may give the gift of sleep and peace of mind to your spouse (or your parent(s)). It may make your children feel safer about your well-being, too. And it may give you more time and energy. What would you do if you had more "spoons" of energy, or another full hour, to spend on a given day? What ripple effect will you be able to have in the world, with less time and energy taken by living with diabetes?

I can't wait to find out what you'll do.

ACKNOWLEDGEMENTS

I wouldn't be where I am today without my parents. Thank you, Mom and Dad, for teaching me to go to the concession stand... and spending several decades telling me to write a book.

I also wouldn't be writing this book without Scott. On our fourth date, we went roller skating. He went to go pull his roller blades out of his trunk, and I asked him why he had a Costco-sized pack of juice boxes in his trunk. "Oh," he said. "I know you said you treat your low BGs with juice boxes and I thought it would be helpful to keep some in my car for you in case you need them while we're out and about." He clearly got it. He got it faster than anyone I've ever met. And he kept asking questions, leading us to realize that teaching him was the same way we could "teach" or instruct a computer to do more heavy lifting in diabetes. And along the way, we fell in love, and he's been with me ever since. Thank you, Scott, for never going "poof" and for so many reasons it would take an entire book to list... but especially being the first

146

round editor of all my writing, including this book!

OpenAPS would not have happened, either, without years of work by Ben West. Thank you, Ben, not only for your years of work on pump communications, and hours spent working with Scott and I on various elements of what became OpenAPS, but also for being an excellent mentor and introducer to open source methodology.

The broader scaling of OpenAPS wouldn't have happened, either, without many of the early adopters of OpenAPS, and all the work they did and continued on to do over the years in various projects in the DIY diabetes community. Continued thanks and hats off to Nate Rackleyft, Pete Schwamb, Chris Hanneman, Mark Wilson, Oskar Pearson, Kevin Lee, John Costik, Jason Calabrese, Sulka Haro, and many, many more.

In an open source community project like OpenAPS, especially ones that grows into a larger community movement, there are hundreds of contributors. People write code, file issues, report bugs, help troubleshoot, document new setups, develop new hardware or software, test things, answer questions,. share their stories, donate their data, and so much more. All of this work is incredibly valuable to the entire community.

Thank you to everyone who has touched, and given so much to, the diabetes community through DIY & open source projects.

And specifically for this book, many thanks to Tim Gunn for front cover design; to Aaron Kowalski for the foreword; as well as to those who provided early feedback and input into the book: Jason Wittmer, Mary Anne Patton, Hamish Crockett, Joanne Dellert, Klara Pickova, Leif Sawyer, Scott Johnson, Sufyan Hussain, Amy Tenderich, Brenda Weedman, Aaron Neinstein.

RESOURCES

Here are some of the resources discussed throughout the book, and other helpful references:

Documentation for a few different DIY diabetes projects:

- Nightscout: https://nightscout.github.io/
- OpenAPS: http://openaps.readthedocs.org/en/latest/
- AndroidAPS:
  https://androidaps.readthedocs.io/en/latest/
- Loop: https://loopkit.github.io/loopdocs/

Related Facebook Groups:

- "Looped" (supports all types of DIY closed loop systems):
  https://www.facebook.com/groups/TheLoopedGroup/
- "CGM In The Cloud" (supports Nightscout-related questions):

https://www.facebook.com/groups/cgminthecloud/

- "CGM In The Cloud Off Topic" (supports all other diabetes-related topics and other tech question): https://www.facebook.com/groups/CGMITCOFFTOPIC/

Research referenced:

- Meta-analysis article (*Tsapas et. al, BMJ*): https://www.bmj.com/content/361/bmj.k1310
- "Excellent Glycemic Control Maintained by Open-Source Hybrid Closed-Loop AndroidAPS During and After Sustained Physical Activity" (*Petruzelkova et al*): https://www.liebertpub.com/doi/10.1089/dia.2018.0214
- "Glycemic Control in Individuals with Type 1 Diabetes Using an Open Source Artificial Pancreas System (OpenAPS)" (*Melmer et al*): https://dom-pubs.onlinelibrary.wiley.com/doi/10.1111/dom.13810
- "Efficacy, safety, and user experience of DIY or open-source artificial pancreas systems: a systematic review" (*Asarani et al*): https://link.springer.com/article/10.1007%2Fs00592-020-01623-4
- "In Silico Trials of an Open-Source Android-Based Artificial Pancreas: A New Paradigm to Test Safety and Efficacy of Do-It-Yourself Systems" (*Toffanin et al*): https://www.liebertpub.com/doi/10.1089/dia.2019.0375

- "A real-world study of user characteristics, safety and efficacy of open-source closed-loop systems and Medtronic 670G" (*Jeyaventhan et al*): https://dom-pubs.onlinelibrary.wiley.com/doi/10.1111/dom.14439?af =R

- "Use of a do-it-yourself artificial pancreas system is associated with better glucose management and higher quality of life among adults with type 1 diabetes" (*Wu et al*):https://journals.sagepub.com/doi/10.1177/204201882 0950146

- "CREATE (Community deRivEd AutomaTEd insulin delivery) trial. Randomised parallel arm open label clinical trial comparing automated insulin delivery using a mobile controller (AnyDANA-loop) with an open-source algorithm with sensor augmented pump therapy in type 1 diabetes" (*Burnside et al*): https://link.springer.com/article/10.1007%2Fs40200-020-00547-8

- All the DIY studies mentioned otherwise are linked from OpenAPS.org/outcomes

Blogs covering living with APS:
- Dana Lewis: https://DIYPS.org/
- Tim Street: http://www.diabettech.com/
- Mary Anne Patton: https://myartificialpancreas.net/

GLOSSARY

Explanations of words, phrases, abbreviations, and acronyms referenced throughout the book:

AndroidAPS - an open source implementation of an APS where the Android phone is the controller and holds a version of the OpenAPS algorithm, and communicates via Bluetooth to a Bluetooth-enabled insulin pump.

APS or AP - Artificial Pancreas System. A term for a closed-loop automated insulin delivery system in which insulin dosing is adjusted to keep or return BG to target.

basal - baseline insulin level that is pre-programmed into your pump and mimics the insulin your pancreas would give throughout the day and night

BG - Blood Glucose

bolus - extra insulin given by a pump, usually to correct for a high Blood Glucose (BG) or for carbohydrates. Differentiated from "basal" or baseline insulin delivery

CGM - Continuous Glucose Monitor, a temporary glucose sensor that is inserted into your skin (with a self-retracting needle) and provides BG readings approximately every 5 minutes. Different models exist in the market with various calibration requirements varying from no calibrations to 2 a day, and official sensor lifetimes varying from 6-10 days.

closed-loop - closed-loop systems make automatic adjustments to basal delivery, without needing user-approval, based on an algorithm. Also known as APS. There are different types, from "hybrid" (where the user is still expected to enter information and manually dose for meals) to "fully" closed loops (where the user does minimal interactions with the system).

carb ratio, or CR - carbohydrate ratio - the amount of carbohydrates that are covered by one standard unit of insulin. Example: 1 U of insulin for 10 carbs.

IOB - Insulin On Board, or insulin active in your body.

Note that most commercially available pumps calculate IOB based on bolus activity only. Some APS may also consider only bolus insulin to be part of IOB. However, the DIY community uses "net" IOB to calculate positive or negative insulin activity relative to your baseline, basal amounts. If evaluating an APS (DIY or commercial), make sure you understand how IOB is calculated.

loop or "looping" - note the lowercase use of this word, meant to describe using a closed loop/APS.

Loop - note the uppercase use of this word, meant to describe one of the DIY systems that holds the algorithm on an iPhone and requires the user to carry a radio device (e.g. "Rileylink") to bridge communications between the pump and the phone.

negative IOB – when your netIOB is less than zero, which can occur when your temporary basal rate adjustments are less than your typically scheduled basal amount at that time. If you frequently get negative IOB at the same time of day on a regular basis, some of your settings may need adjusting.

net IOB - amount of Insulin On Board, taking into account any adjusted (higher or lower) basal rates (see basal IOB above) plus bolus activity.

NS, or Nightscout - a cloud-based visualization and remote-monitoring tool, designed by and for the diabetes community.

OpenAPS - refers to the open source artificial pancreas movement, as well as a specific DIY system. An OpenAPS system has a small computer controller, a "rig", that holds the algorithm and has a radio to communicate with the insulin pump and CGM.

open loop - open-loop systems will suggest recommended adjustments to insulin dosing, but will not enact those suggestions. It's a decision support system, but not a closed loop.

oref0 - another name for the main algorithm used in OpenAPS

Time in Range (TIR) – a newer, standardized way of reporting CGM data, in addition to the A1c metric. Typical TIR for research studies is a range from 80-180 mg/dL, although different studies and different individuals may report or strive for different ranges.

ABOUT THE AUTHOR

Dana M. Lewis is one of the creators and founders of the Open Source Artificial Pancreas System (OpenAPS), and is passionate about increasing access and availability of artificial pancreas technology globally. She's spent 8 years writing dozens of blog posts about first-hand experiences and has numerous peer-reviewed papers aggregating data from the DIY community and documenting how to further improve DIY and commercial closed loop systems.